Dual diagnosis: filling the gap

ISBN 2-7420-0500-5

Éditions John Libbey Eurotext
127, avenue de la République, 92120 Montrouge, France
Tél. : 01 46 73 06 60
E-mail : contact@john-libbey-eurotext.fr
Site internet : http://www.john-libbey-eurotext.fr

John Libbey Eurotext
42-46 High Street
Esher, Surrey
KT10 9KY
United Kingdom

CIC Edizioni Internazionali
Corso Trieste 42
00198 Roma, Italia
Tel. : (39) 06 841 26 73

© 2003, John Libbey Eurotext, Paris

Il est interdit de reproduire intégralement ou partiellement le présent ouvrage sans autorisation de l'éditeur ou du Centre Français d'Exploitation du Droit de Copie, 20, rue des Grands-Augustins, 75006 Paris.

Italian Association on Addiction Psychiatry
2002 International Meeting Proceedings

Dual diagnosis: filling the gap

Edited by

Giuseppe Carrà and Massimo Clerici

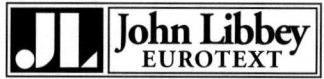

M. T. Abou-Saleh
A. Arteman
A. Blasi
L. M.C. van den Bosch
W. van den Brink
E. Bruguera
G. Carrà
M. Casas
M. Clerici
F. Collazos
P. Duro
G. Escuder
A. Gual
M. Krausz
A. Lowe
P. Lusilla
G. Mammana
V. Marcos
M. Martinez
M. Martone
J. Matali
A.T. McLellan
K. Nicolaou
A. Öjehagen
J. Padrós
A. Ramos
C. Roncero
I. Schaar
G. M. Schippers
G. Sestini
R. Verheul

Contents

Prefaces
G. Sestini, M. Martone, G. Mammana.. VII

Introduction
M. Clerici, G. Carrà.. 1

Is Addiction an illness – Can it be treated?
A. T. McLellan.. 3

The British experience of dual diagnosis in the national health service
A. Lowe, M. T. Abou-Saleh... 41

Mentally ill substance abusers in Sweden. A 5-year follow-up of a multisite study of co-operation between psychiatric services and social authorities
A. Öjehagen, I. Schaar.. 49

Heroin assisted treatment of drug addicts
M. Krausz... 55

Treatment system and intervention strategies for mentally ill substance abusers: the Greek experience
K. Nicolaou 61

Dialectical behavior therapy of borderline patients with and without substance use problems: implementation and long term effects
L. M.C. van den Bosch, R. Verheul, G. M. Schippers, W. von den Brink............................. 67

The integral care programme for sick physicians (PAIMM) of the medical council of Barcelona
P. Lusilla, E. Bruguera, A. Arteman, A. Gual, M. Martínez, V. Marcos, G. Escuder, J. Matalí, C. Roncero, A. Ramos, F. Collazos, P. Duro, A. Blasi, J. Padrós, M. Casas 77

36-month follow up of opiate dependents in three levels of treatment intensity
M. Clerici, G. Carrà.. 85

Prefaces

Those who are daily confronted with the problem of substance abuse are always puzzled by the personality of those who have become abusers, by their frequent relapses and failures and by the great difficulties encountered working in this field.

One of the reasons for such difficulties is, no doubt, linked to the presence of psychiatric disturbances that, in some cases precede and, in some other cases are either concurrent or subsequent to substance use, abuse and dependence. The evidence-based co-presence of substance abuse and psychiatric problems has been referred to as psychiatric comorbidity for some years now. This means that sometimes important psychiatric problems are present in the subject before he/she starts to make use of substances and that these problems will not necessarily be related to the use of substances. Or, the same term psychiatric comorbidity may refer to the pathogenic effects of the abused substances on the central nervous system of the abuser as these substances are not inert substances once they reach our nervous system.

Some of these behavioural changes remain more or less irreversible once the substance abuse ends, even if scientific research in this field remains full of gaps. This raises very important questions, not only in terms of the treatment or rehabilitation of substance abusers, but also in terms of what a policymaker could do to speed up the solution of these problems by improving the comprehensive quality of the measures to be taken in this field.

It is for this very reason that, on the occasion of the six months of the Italian Presidency of the European Union, the Ministry of Work and Social Policies has focused its attention on the topic of both the diagnosis and co-occurrence of psychiatric disorders and substance abuse. A more in-depth study of this matter and the contributions of experts are likely to help us provide political and administrative indications to tackle the problem when it emerges.

These suggestions are intended to help us improve our present responses to substance abuse treatment.

Senator Grazia Sestini
Vice minister, Italian Ministry of Work and Social Policies

The General Direction of the Observatory on Substance and Alcohol Abuse is an administrative body that represents the arm of the Ministry of Work and Social Policies for its actions in the field of substance abuse.

Currently the Italian Ministry of Work and Social Policies avails itself of an Observatory on Substance Abuse that collects all the epidemiological data coming from various other Ministries and works out an annual report on the state of substance abuse in Italy to be submitted to the Parliament.

The Substance Abuse Observatory has it own Scientific Board made of eight experts that supervise and define the objectives of the activities of the Observatory itself and indicate the technical and scientific orientations for the action.

This General Direction also hosts a National Scientific Committee of experts of substance abuse where the operators of both public and private services are represented together with representatives of the associations of substance abusers' families and of the other Ministries operating in this field.

Finally, the Ministry of Work and Social Policies is assigned a national fund for the control of drug abuse. 75% of this fund is allocated to Regional Boards and 25% is under direct management of the Ministry for its National Action Plans.

Every year a Call for Bids is launched which gives public and private agencies the possibility to submit nation-wide projects in the field of substance abuse.

Also the guidelines for the allocation of funds to these projects have currently been defined.

In the last few years the problem of psychiatric comorbidity has acquired a growing importance drawing the attention of both the Observatory and its Scientific Board and of the people in charge of the projects likely to be funded with the national fund fo the control of drug abuse.

This is the reason why it was decided to assign to this topic an important session of the Conference on Substance Abuse that our Ministry has organized within the Italian Six-Months Presidency of the European Union.

These materials are intended to inspire our technical and administrative work in this sensitive matter.

Mariano Martone
General director addiction and observatory substance abuse and alcoholism,
Ministry of Work and Social Policies

The problem of dual diagnosis and comorbidity that often exists in terms of the effects of substance use and abuse on the mind and the evidence of other psychiatric disturbances, falling within DSM IV classification, represents a topic that attracts a growing attention on the part of the clinicians who work in the field of substance abuse.

In this field a shift has been registered from ignoring and fully repressing the problem – an attitude that has characterized in the last twenty years, with few laudable exceptions, the clinical approach to pathological dependence – to the often a critical consideration of this phenomenon as one of the many problems of modern society.

Nowadays the most varied behaviours are observed in this field which essentially consist of a sort of self-attributed competence in this "new discipline" (dual diagnosis) that does not imply any kinds of modification in our way of operating.

Dual diagnosis seems to be often utilized to confirm the sometimes iatrogenic cronicization and adaptation of the patients to a frequently remissive clinical practice which remains heavily dependent on the administration of drugs meant to replace the substance and poor in terms of innovative tools and resources that could stimulate the recovery of the patients.

We believe that the issue of dual diagnosis is an issue of utmost importance in our clinical and educational fields and that, just for this very reason, it cannot be either underevaluated or exploited for second thoughts. Quite the contrary, dual diagnosis accounts for a fundamental occasion for a critical review of the clinical and educational understanding of the pathology we are concerned with as well as for changing the responses that today we give to substance abusers in terms of both clinical practice and education.

In this respect the topic of diagnosis should, first of all, be revised.

Actually we speak of dual diagnosis but in Italian services it is very often impossible even to speak of a diagnosis as the identification of the case relies in most cases on only one criterion *i.e.* having made use of substances, and does not take into account any other piece of knowledge on the personality the drug abuser and of the dynamics of this personality within his/her behaviours other than drug abuse.

A first serious step ahead we should take in this direction should be represented by an attempt to define commonly recognized serious diagnostic criteria intended to formulate a multidisciplinary and multi-axial diagnosis.

But a correct framing of the cases according to correct criteria cannot fail to consider two steps that are crucial to us:

– Critical observation of drug abuse in active conditions (while he/she makes use of substances) and in drug-free conditions in a protected environment.

Such observation needs a dynamic dimension as it does not enable to formulate a diagnosis "in one morning", but rather over medium, long periods during which the drug-free conditions may let pre-existing mental disturbances or substance-induced disorders emerge. The treatment of these same disturbances can be modified over time thus modifying the same clinical picture. Dynamic diagnosis should be permitted to take place from the time of the first intake onwards. For this reason dynamic diagnosis calls for a common approach and spirit on the part of the different wards and services that collaborate in the treatment of substance abusers.

Such common spirit and approach based on the observation of the treatment in different settings, calls for an integrated training of the operators of the different wards and services.

On these foundations a useful monitoring of the treatment destined to substance abusers can be established in a later phase.

- The availability of diagnostic tools that have to be used by the operators participating in the therapeutical process at different levels and to define both the complex clinical condition of the substance abuser and the possible co-presence of psychiatric disturbances. These tools include, of course, ASI, SCID, MMPI, but the real problem is how to put in place a tangible diagnostic procedure useful and easy to be implemented that takes into account the reality of our services as well as their necessary involvement in this procedure.

An accurate diagnosis is expected to uncover, as shown by the international scientific literature, the co-presence, with different prevalence rates, of substance-induced disturbances and of psychotic personality and mood disorders.

Of course, these are completely different conditions from both the point of view of diagnosis and, most importantly, of treatment.

As to this latter point of view, as is the case for psychiatry, some low – average – and high – psychiatric intensity conditions could occur.

Now, taking into account this situation could be useful to define the standards required for the personnel and the facilities expected to take care of these cases.

Such a new organization of the rehabilitation facilities would allow for keeping a right balance between clinical and educational functions. This balance is not only necessary for the treatment of this pathology, but it also respects the story of these services as it has been constructed over time. This is even more true for the diverse European ways to cope with this problem.

In the absence of this balance we would continue to feed the present situation of chaos where we fluctuate from a hypocritical misknowledge of the problem to magic self-attributed competence.

Also the problem of relapse and of its prevention would be given another dimension and importance in a perspective of a greater, albeit non disproportionate, consideration of the issue of the dual diagnosis. How could we explain the high rate of relapses in the field of substance abuse if not as the outcome of very frequent misdiagnoses that are not even formulated or are formulated once the clinical picture has worsened or become chronic also because of confused and inefficient interventions? A dynamic diagnosis of the individual cases in the different phases of treatment would allow for a better clinical awareness and for ready to be modified and verified treatments. Anyhow in case of relapse we would – maybe – be able to give a name to the condition treating and preventing it as far as we can.

The issue of the possible, or sometimes, impossible reintegration of the substance abuser with psychiatric comorbidity of different levels into the work world would be talked in a completely different manner.

If it is true that a certain percentage of substance abusers are affected by serious mental disorders, we cannot understand why their conditions are seldom assessed in terms of their ability to work as is the case for psychiatric patients for whom it is much easier to get disability pensions or recognition of reduced professional skills.

Of course this path may be full of enormous obstacles linked to the natural predisposition of those who exhibit a personality and a behaviour that lead to pathologically dependent attitudes in each and every aspects of their lives, work included. The tangible risk does exist that this may become a channel of free privileges and not a guarantee of rights for really sick people.

Nevertheless a serious reflection on what a good diagnosis could do to improve the condition of our patients, at least the most serious and elderly of our patients, cannot be postponed any longer now that we are aware of the presence, in some cases, of important problems of psychiatric comorbidity.

In the face of the growing likelihood of comorbidities, we have to talk the problem of who is going to make the diagnosis and of the professional background this person has to possess.

Once again the problem emerges of the personnel who operate in the public and private services and of their training in the use of recognized and validated diagnostic tools employed in the services where they work. As these services have met over the years and still continue to meet the needs of a massive population of substance abusers made by now of a large number of people of different generations who also need psychiatric treatment, time has come to define new specific professional profiles to be added to the traditional ones of the physician, psychologist, and social worker. A new speciality in this field could be established to respond to the needs of these new professional profiles (why we should not think of a pathological dependence technician) and also a Master Course to be followed after having obtained the traditional university degrees could be set up.

In this case the possibility of improving the diagnostic skills of the personnel working in these services does not seem to be attainable without revising the objectives and methods of functioning of the same and without appropriate investments in the training and requalification of the existing personnel.

Finally, there is the problem of the costs to incur to formulate a dual diagnosis and pay the relevant treatment.

It is our belief that, in general, the "system" of substance abuse should do a great effort to develop the fields of diagnosis, treatment monitoring and scientific research to supplement its merely clinical and educational activities.

This raises the issues of the costs that the European Union member states should bear in their fight against an evil that may be come a scourge for the young European generations.

For this reason it has been our intention to provide the participants in the Cagliari Round Table with this scientific paper that is intended to lay the foundations of new and clear actions in the field of dual diagnosis.

Giuseppe Mammana
Italian representative management board, OETD Lisbon

Introduction

The treatment of co-morbidity, that is the concurrence of substance abuse issues with psychiatric disorders, has assumed great relevance for epidemiological, clinical and management concerns and necessitates changes in treatment strategy organization.

In a broad sense, in Italy, the area of drug related problems research has developed slowly and suffers from operative limitations in comparison with other European countries that have a more integrated approach and a strong chemical dependency treatment development.

The "diversity" of the Italian approach can be explained in historical terms. Our nation, despite having a virtually unrivalled medical care system worldwide with one of the highest numbers of health-care professionals, has produced little clinical-epidemiological research in this field. On the health-care management plane, there is a gap between the mental health care system and drug-dependency care.

This gap manifests itself among health-care services within different therapy and organisational systems, and in the position of the private Therapeutic Community in the system of addiction treatment in Italy.

Related to this is the vicarious role that the constellation of therapeutic communities has had in Italy with respect to the system of public services up until the end of the 1980s. In many regions specific criteria for accreditation of private health care structures have only recently been defined.

Meanwhile, the public health system for addictions has changed from a focus on outpatient services to having a departmentalized structure. It manages different operational units, plans treatment, care and prevention programs, and interfaces with other departments, mainly mental health, which concur to the care of patients with complex needs.

The differences between Italian and European health care are decreasing in terms of availability of professional management oriented care with quality and cost controls and in terms of a stronger commitment to assessment, structured diagnoses, monitored courses of therapy and measurement of treatment efficacy.

Some of these objectives have come up against criticism, rigidity in the system, difficulties in absorbing and valuing differing competencies and serious limits in acquiring funding. The current debate on political and administrative levels can doubtless contribute to accelerating change and reducing the current obstacles.

This approach to the issue of psychiatric co-morbidity in substance abusers, also known as "dual diagnosis", is a reality of health-care management that varies greatly from nation to nation.

The shape given to the management of this phenomenon currently takes a psychiatric focus (US Model) or a generalist concept that attributes competencies and resources, reinforcing primary care (European model), or finally a concept of specialized services separate enough from different disciplines. It deals more with selected patients or privileged health-issue areas rather than belonging to a specific health service system.

With such complexity of solutions, it is either health or care management orientations that create the pivot. We consider these orientations responsible for the finding and removal of funding that "maintains" the system and the redistribution of patients' cost load, which inevitably falls to the margins of various service systems: specialized medicine, psychiatry, drug-dependency not to mention others!

Given this, the choice among a public health-care system, a totally private system (especially if insurance-based) or a mixed system (public-private accredited profit or public-private nonprofit, accredited or less) complicates our ability to understand individual experiences, complex system functions, and especially the results that this work makes available.

These days, such comparative work is based on epidemiological data, diagnosis and treatment, and mid to long-term follow-up research. It is also a valuable resource for assessment protocol management and the creation of operative guidelines.

The creation and maintenance of initiatives to understand these themes along with multi-centric, possibly longitudinal, research perhaps can offer relevant contributions to the reciprocal knowledge among health-care professionals from different countries. This can help create a professional European health-care system.

This volume springs from the need to improve knowledge among health-care professionals from various countries and to create a common set of qualifications among different therapeutic care systems.

The Italian Association on Addiction Psychiatry (SIP.Dip) has been actively involved in a greater understanding and openness toward the differing situations in other countries ever since it was established as a Special Section of the Italian Psychiatric Association (SIP) in 1989. The related International framework refers to the Section on Alcoholism and Drug Addiction of the Association of European Psychiatrists – AEP, coordinated by Mats Berglund and to the Section on Addiction Psychiatry of the World Psychiatry Association – WPA, coordinated by Nady El-Guebaly. In concert, these Associations have been able to offer more and more propositions on their common theme and continued professional and scientific training for Italian health-care professionals who work between psychiatry and addiction fields. This volume is a wide-spectrum reflection springing from the contributions of some of the most important European and American researchers in the dual diagnosis field, who were involved in the national SIP.Dip. Conference in Milan July 2002. They contributed to a shared understanding of issues such as the relevance of psychiatric diagnosis in addiction treatment planning, with experiences from Germany, Netherlands, Greece, Spain, England, Italy and Thomas McLellan's paradigmatic research on assessment instruments carried out over the last 30 years in the USA.

With this volume's publication, our association is proud to spread international points of view in the National and European fields. We intend to continue to work with cultural and scientific events to the benefit of professionals in the Italian health-care system in conjunction with national projects and policies at various levels.

Massimo Clerici and Giuseppe Carrà
Milan October 16th, 2003

Is Addiction an illness – Can it be treated?*

A. T. McLellan

The Treatment Research Institute at the Penn – VA Center for Studies of Addiction, Phila. Pa.

Problems of alcohol and drug dependence produce dramatic costs to society in terms of lost productivity, social disorder and of course health care utilization [1, 2]. One recent study [3] estimated that alcohol abuse and dependence cost society approximately $90 billion and that abuse of other drugs cost approximately $67 billion each year. A recent study funded by the Robert Wood Johnson Foundation reported over 1/4 of all deaths in this country were associated in some way with alcohol, drug or tobacco use [4]. Perhaps more subtle but no less significant is the fact that more than three fourths of all foster children in this country are the products of alcohol and/or drug dependent parents [5]. In response to this threat to the general welfare, there has been renewed interest in the development and expansion of treatment programs as a method of dealing with these substance abuse problems. Yet, while some segments of the public are demanding greater availability and more financing for substance dependence treatments, there are those in government, insurance, managed care and the public who question the efficacy of these treatments, and whether they are "worth it" [6]. As recently as 1997, the *Wall Street* Journal questioned the effectiveness and value of substance abuse treatment, saying "... The success rate of treatment programs is highly uncertain" [7].

The negative opinions about the effectiveness and value of substance abuse treatment appear to relate to core public perceptions about addiction and about what would be an "effective" addiction intervention, regardless of the type of intervention. The first perception is that drug addiction is primarily a "social problem" requiring a social-judicial remedy – rather than a "health problem" requiring prevention and treatment. This perception is quite understandable given the relative prominence of the social problems caused by drug and alcohol abuse. Crime, family disruption, loss of economic productivity and social decay are the most observable, dangerous and expensive effects of drugs on the social systems of our country. Thus, it is not surprising that many in the legislature and in the public at large expect law enforcement and interdiction efforts instead of public health efforts to correct the "drug problem".

Other important perceptions in this area involve widespread scepticism about the advisability, effectiveness and value of treatments for addiction. For example, many individuals believe that a medical or treatment-oriented approach to substance abuse conveys uncomfortable implicit messages. For example, some believe that to call addiction an illness suggests that the addicted person is not responsible for the addiction – nor the addiction-related problems; that they "can't

---

* Supported by the National Institute on Drug Abuse, the Center for Substance Abuse Treatment, the Office of National Drug Control Policy, the Department of Veterans Affairs and the Robert Wood Johnson Foundation.

help themselves". These are messages that many people find offensive and unfair. There is also the pervasive view that treatments are designed to help the drug user – but *not* designed to help society. Why should a society expend public resources to help individuals who may have produced many social problems? Finally, many in the public do not believe that treatment "works". Specifically, many do not believe that any treatment can get addicted persons "off drugs and alcohol" and *keep* them off [7].

This is a view that is apparently shared by many physicians. Few medical schools have an adequate required course in addiction. It has been repeatedly documented over the past three decades that a majority of physicians do not screen for signs of alcohol or drug dependence during routine examinations [8, 9]. Apparently there is the feeling that such screening efforts are wasted since in a 1997 survey, a majority of general practise physicians and nurses indicated that none of the currently available medical or health care interventions would be appropriate or effective in treating addiction [10].

It is well known that many persons who have received treatments have returned to alcohol and drug use. This "failure" of substance abuse treatments to reliably produce longstanding abstinence is seen as confirming the suspicions about treatment held by many Americans. Thus, treatment interventions that admittedly cannot cure the addiction and that may be seen as focusing only on helping an addicted individual – at great cost to society – are not widely popular. But are these perceptions true? Is there a role for addiction treatment in public policy aimed at reducing demand for drugs and reducing the social harms and costs associated with drug abuse? If treatments were considered a wise public investment, what treatments – behavioural interventions, medications or combinations – should be provided. Finally, is there evidence that these addiction treatments can be effective and valuable – not just to the affected patient – but to the society that would be expected to support those treatments?

In the text that follows we consider these questions from several perspectives. In *Part I* we ask whether there is evidence to suggest that addiction could be an illness:

- Is it possible to reliably diagnose "dependence" or "addiction" and to differentiate it from simple "drug use"?
- Is there a predictable onset and course to the addictive disorders?
- Is there evidence for genetic heritability in the susceptibility to addictive disorders?
- And are there brain and physiological changes associated with the progression from drug use to addiction – and how long do these changes last*?

Thus, in *Part II* of the paper, we examine the evidence basis for recently developed medications and medically oriented behavioural interventions. Here we address the question of whether there is evidence that medically oriented treatments for addiction could be effective and valuable to a society, relative to these other social policy alternatives – and whether incarceration and other forms of criminal justice interventions could be effectively combined with treatments.

In *Part III* of the paper we review the available research on specific treatment processes and treatment components that may be the "active ingredients" in effective drug abuse treatment. This review covers the past fifteen years and includes only data from clinical trials, treatment matching program studies, or health services studies where the patients were adults who were clearly alcohol or drug (excluding tobacco) dependent by contemporary criteria, where the treatment provided was a conventional form of rehabilitation (any setting or modality), and where there were measures of treatment processes and post-treatment outcome.

---

* It is important to acknowledge at the outset that even substantial evidence in these areas will not *prove* that addiction is an illness. Such evidence will only suggest that the onset, course and presentation parameters seen in addiction are *similar* to those same parameters in other diseases. Moreover, it is also clear that even if we were able in some way to prove that addiction were an illness – it is an entirely separate but equally important question whether currently available medical interventions would be effective in addressing addiction problems.

In *Part IV* of the paper we consider why it appears that addiction treatment is not as potent or effective as treatments for other medical disorders. To inform and frame this discussion we compare addiction treatments with treatments for three well-studied, chronic medical illnesses – adult onset hypertension, diabetes and asthma. The examination of this issue leads to particularly important conclusions regarding how addiction treatment is conceptualized by the public, how it is typically provided by treatment programs and how it has been evaluated by researchers. Here we suggest how addiction might be treated, insured and evaluated if it were considered a chronic illness.

■ Part 1. Is addiction an illness: how could you know?

There has been much debate regarding the inappropriate "medicalization" of various conditions and problems [11]. The public has grown skeptical of new "syndromes" and conditions that do not appear to conform to common sense diagnostic criteria for "true" medical illnesses; or of "conditions" that have no known treatments. For example, a recent New York Times editorial [12] suggests that to consider cigarette smoking a medical disorder "... shifts responsibility away from the individual...", helps doctors profit, and has "... Little to do with improving the public health". In this context, many believe that "medicalization" of addiction is simply a way for physicians to declare more territory under their jurisdiction. Much of this scepticism is understandable when the term addiction has been applied to sex, gambling, work and even chocolate. Given this background it is reasonable to ask how any "condition" comes to be considered a "medical illness" [11]. Here, we have tried to apply the same standards and methods that are currently used in the study of aetiology, diagnosis and course of other disorders (*e.g.* diabetes, asthma, hypertension, etc.) to the study of drug dependence.

Advances in Diagnosing Drug Dependence

Perhaps the first question a physician might ask to determine whether a presenting "condition" is actually a medical disorder, is whether the supposed pathologic "illness" can be reliably differentiated from a non-pathologic state. This contrast has not always been clear in the area of alcohol and drug dependence, due in part to the fact that most adults have "used" alcohol and/or other drugs during their lives – sometimes heavily to the point of "abuse" – but rarely to the point where it could reasonably be called an "illness".

Further compounding this difficulty has been the lack of a laboratory test for "dependence" or even standardized definitions for the terms "addiction" and "dependence". The vagueness of these terms meant that diagnoses were often unreliable across different practitioners or different parts of the country. This situation has changed dramatically as a result of the concept of the dependence syndrome formulated by Edwards and Gross [13] and translated operationally through the Diagnostic and Statistical Manual of Mental Disorders (the DSM) [14]. In the current edition (fourth) of the DSM, "dependence" is defined as a pathologic condition that is manifest by a "... Compulsive desire for the drug (or drugs) despite serious adverse consequences" [14].

There are seven specific diagnostic criteria that a practitioner must consider in making a DSM diagnosis of dependence and three or more of these must be satisfied for a valid diagnosis of dependence. Two of these criteria – tolerance and withdrawal – are considered evidence of neurological and behavioural adaptation to a drug. Tolerance is operationalized in the criteria through evidence that "... Greater quantities must be used to produce the same effect..." [14]. Withdrawal is evidenced by physical signs indicating "... A syndrome of an unpleasant and often dangerous health condition developing hours to days following the cessation of the drug use..." [14]. While tolerance and withdrawal had been cardinal features of drugs such as nicotine, alcohol, opioids, benzodiazepines and barbiturates for many years, there has been recent evidence for tolerance and withdrawal associated with tetrahydro cannabinol (THC) the most prominent active ingredient in marijuana [15, 16].

Additional DSM criteria inquire about whether a patient has "... reduced or eliminated previously pleasurable activities in order to concentrate on obtaining the substance..." and whether the patient has "... used the substance instead of or while performing important responsibilities or functions..." [14]. Answers to these seven diagnostic questions have been found to be more sensitive and specific than many laboratory tests used in diagnosing other illnesses such as prostate and breast cancers [17].

Genetic Factors in Drug Dependence

While many diseases are not genetically transmitted (*e.g.* Tuberculosis) and many heritable traits are not diseases (*e.g.* eye colour), genetic transmission is one of the many criteria that a physician might use to decide whether a presenting "condition" is a medical illness. In this regard, Rounsaville *et al.* [18, 19] used standard diagnostic criteria to examine rates of alcoholism and drug dependence in the general population and among family members of diagnosed alcohol and drug dependent individuals. They found prevalence rates of approximately 11% for alcoholism and 6% for any type of other drug dependence in the general population. This compared with rates of 38% for alcoholism and 41% for drug dependence in family members of diagnosed alcohol or drug dependent individuals. In a separate study of siblings of diagnosed drug dependent individuals, 92% who tried a drug went on to meet diagnostic criteria for dependence [19]. This compared with only an 18% rate of drug dependence among siblings of non-drug dependent individuals who tried the same drugs.

While these studies suggest that drug dependence "runs in families", many factors are known to operate in "familial transmission" and direct genetic heritability is only one of these. One of the best methods to estimate the level of genetic contribution within all the cultural and environmental variables that are operational in familial transmission is to examine the relative rates of a disorder in monozygotic and dizygotic twins. For example, heritability estimates (H^2) from twin studies of hypertension range from .25-.50 depending upon the sample and the diagnostic criteria used [20-22]. Similarly, twin studies of diabetes offer heritability estimates of approximately .80 for type 1 (insulin dependent) [23] to about .30-.55 for type 2 (non insulin dependent) diabetes [24]. Finally, twin studies of adult onset asthma have produced a somewhat broader range of heritability estimates, ranging from .36 to .70 [25, 26].

In the addiction field, four twin studies have been published over the past five years [27-30] and all found significantly higher rates of alcoholism and/or drug dependence among twins than among siblings and higher rates among monozygotic than dizygotic twin pairs. A recent twin study of heroin dependence produced a heritability estimate of .34 among males [28]. Similar studies of alcohol dependence have produced heritability estimates of .55 to .65 among males [29, 31]. Though there are still very few studies of heritability in the field of addiction and there is a need for studies of specific heritabilities by substance and by gender, the evidence accumulated over the past few years suggests significant contribution of genetic influence in approximately the same range as for chronic illnesses such as asthma and hypertension.

Comparing the factors associated with the onset and course of illness in drug dependence and other illnesses

The evidence presented thus far suggests that drug dependence can be reliably and validly diagnosed and that there is evidence of genetic (as well as familial) transmission associated with contracting the illness. However, since the use of these substances is, at least initially, a voluntary action, behavioural control or "will power" is obviously a very important factor in the onset of these addictive disorders. At some level, and particularly in the case of dependence on illegal substances, the addicted individual is "at fault" for initiating the behaviors that later combine with the social, environmental and genetic factors to produce the dependence disorder. Though an addicted person may have been genetically predisposed to contract the illness and may have been raised in an environment that contained known risk factors, it remains a fact that this individual's behavioural choices played a prominent role in the onset and course of the disorder. Doesn't this voluntary initiation of the "disease process" set drug dependence apart, etiologically, from other medical illnesses?

In fact, there are many illness where "voluntary choice" contributes significantly to initiate and sustain a disease process – especially when these voluntary behaviors interact with genetic and cultural factors. For example, there is clear evidence, at least among males, that "salt sensitivity" is genetically transmitted (heritability estimate is .74) [32, 33] and salt sensitivity is a known risk factor for the eventual development of at least one form of hypertension. However, not all of those who inherit salt sensitivity go on to develop hypertension. This is because the *use of salt* is much more likely to be determined by familial salt use patterns, cultural factors and individual choice. Similarly, factors such as obesity, stress level, and exercise are the joint product of familial, cultural, environmental and personal choice factors [30-32]. Thus, while a diabetic, hypertensive or asthmatic patient may have been genetically predisposed to contract a disorder; and may have been raised in an environment that contained known risk factors such as poor parenting, poor diet, smoking and high stress, it is also true that behavioural choices such as the ingestion of high sugar and/or high cholesterol foods, smoking and failure to exercise, also played a role in the onset and severity of their disorder.

There is another aspect to the issue of voluntary choice as a contributor to the initiation of a disease process. This is the role of *involuntary* components embedded within seemingly volitional choices. For example, although the choice to try a drug the first time appears to be completely voluntary, it can be influenced by uncontrolled cultural, economic and ecological factors such as peer pressure, price, and especially availability, that are not completely determined by individual choice. For example, none of our grandmothers had the choice to use "crack" cocaine, ecstasy, GHB or LSD. In contrast, many children today are regularly offered these choices with substantial external pressures.

Further, it is clear that only a small minority of those who make the bad choice to use alcohol or another drug go on to develop addiction. Is this merely evidence that some people are "weak willed" while others "come to their senses"? In fact, the effects of the initial sampling of a drug are also influenced by genetic heritability and in turn are likely to modify the course of continued use in an *involuntary* manner. Those whose initial physiological response to alcohol or other drugs is extremely pleasurable may be more likely to repeat the drug-taking than those whose involuntary, physiological reaction is neutral or even negative. Work by Schuckit et al. with sons of alcohol dependent fathers has shown that these sons are born with more tolerance to alcohol's effects than sons of non alcohol dependent fathers and that this effect is highly influenced by direct genetic transmission (heritability estimate is .67) [34, 35]. Thus the positive effects of alcohol that may be experienced at relatively low doses by most individuals may only be experienced at higher doses by sons of alcohol dependent fathers. In turn, the negative, "hangover" effects of alcohol that may be felt by sons of normal fathers may not be experienced at the same level by sons of alcohol dependent fathers.

In contrast, an example of inherited "supersensitivity" to alcohol has been shown in a large proportion of Chinese and Japanese individuals who experience an involuntary skin "flushing" response to alcohol. This effect has been traced to the presence of an aldehyde dehydrogenase gene that controls a central part of alcohol metabolism [36-38]. Individuals who are homozygous for this allele (approximately 35% of Chinese population), have an especially unpleasant reaction to alcohol. This negative reaction reduces the appeal of alcohol to the point where there have been no alcoholics found with this genotype [36].

For those who do not have an initially negative reaction to their first drug administration, continued repetition of "voluntary" drug taking begins to change – often imperceptibly – into "involuntary" drug taking, ultimately to the point where the behavior is driven by a compulsive craving for the drug. In the text that follows we explore the physiological and molecular bases for these changes.

Pathophysiology Associated with Drug Dependence

The evidence presented thus far suggests that drug dependence has many of the elements of onset and presentation that are exhibited by other illnesses. However, it is a separate question whether there is a predictable pattern of pathophysiological changes such as those generally seen in the course of other medical illnesses. How does the voluntary choice to use alcohol or another drug ultimately become an involuntary compulsion? In fact, the acute effects of alcohol and many other drugs have been well characterized for many years. But even a complete understanding of these acute effects is inadequate to address fundamental questions regarding the mechanisms by which repeated doses of alcohol and other drugs produce paradoxically *increasing* tolerance to the effects of those drugs concurrent with *decreasing* volitional ability to forego the drug. As suggested by Koob and Bloom [39], the challenge is to find an internally consistent sequence by which molecular events modify cellular events, and in turn produce profound and lasting changes in cognitions, motivation and behavior.

Research in the neurochemical, neuroendocrine and cellular changes associated with drug dependence has led literally to volumes of remarkable findings over the past decade. These advances have been summarized in recent special issues of *Science* [40] and *Lancet* [41] and in two volumes produced by the Institute of Medicine of the National Academy of Sciences [42, 43]. Here we will summarize just three areas of investigation that have produced clinically relevant information leading to medications to treat drug dependence.

There is now clear evidence that most addictive drugs have well specified effects on the brain circuitry that is involved in the control of motivated and learned behaviors. This evidence originated from studies in animals [42-44], and with recent developments in brain imaging techniques, has been confirmed in humans [45, 46]. Anatomically, the brain circuitry principally involved in most of the actions of the major addictive drugs is the ventral tegmental area connecting the limbic cortex through the midbrain, to the nucleus accumbens [39, 47]. Neurochemically, all of the major drugs of abuse (alcohol, opiates, cocaine, nicotine) have significant effects on the dopamine system – although through different mechanisms. For example, cocaine increases synaptic dopamine by blocking re-uptake into the pre-synaptic neuron; amphetamine produces increased pre-synaptic release of dopamine, while opiates and alcohol disinhibit dopamine neurons thereby producing increased firing rates [39-44].

Opiates and alcohol also have a direct effect on the endogenous opioid system [39-44]. This finding has led directly to the development and wide clinical use of four effective medications (see below). Evidence is also emerging that the GABA system plays a central role in alcohol dependence and again, this has led to the development of an effective medication to treat alcohol dependence (see below). Finally, recent work on the stress response system suggests the possibility that lasting changes in neurochemical and neuroendocrine function may occur with the development of cocaine and/or opiate dependence [48, 49].

Significantly, the ventral tegmental area and the dopamine system are part of what have been called "survival circuitry" that accounts for some of our most basic behaviors including feeding, flight or fight responses in dangerous situations and sexual behavior. These brain areas have also been associated with the feelings of euphoria produced by naturally occurring reinforcers such as food, sleep and sex [50, 51]. In experiments, animals who receive mild electrical stimulation of the dopamine system contingent upon a lever press response, will rapidly learn to press that lever tens of thousands of times, ignoring normal needs for water, food or rest, in order to maintain the stimulation of that system [43]. Cocaine, opiates and several other dependence producing drugs stimulate this reward circuitry in a supernormal manner [47] producing extremely powerful reward sensations. It is not hard to understand how addictive drugs can produce an immediate and profound desire for their readministration. What is less clear is why simply preventing the administration of these drugs for some period of time (for example, by "detoxifying" the addict or locking them in jail) would not correct the situation, set the system back to normal and, like the child who burned his fingers, lead to a "sadder but wiser" individual who would be less (instead of more) likely to readminister those drugs.

Two explanations seem possible from the research done thus far. The most direct answer is that use of a drug at some dose, frequency and chronicity will reliably produce enduring and possibly permanent pathophysiological changes in the reward circuitry [43, 51, 52], in the "normal" levels of many neurochemicals [52-54] and to the stress response system [51, 52]. It is not clear just how much drug use is required to create these changes, how enduring the various effects are, or whether these effects will ever return to "normal". Physical signs of withdrawal generally last several days, motivational symptoms of withdrawal and cognitive impairment may last several months [43] and the learned aspects of tolerance to the drug may never return to normal [45, 46, 55]. For example, Volkow found impairments in the dopamine system (reduced D2 binding) of abstinent former cocaine users for as long as three months after their last cocaine use [52, 53]. In addition, her research team found reduced glucose metabolism in dopamine projection areas during cocaine abstinence [54], and the degree of metabolism reduction correlated with the long-term reductions in radioligand binding [53]. Another human imaging study found decreased uptake of radiolabled DOPA into the striatum of cocaine users tested one week after their last cocaine dose, indicating decreased dopamine synthesis at this early time point [56]. Still other studies have documented areas of poor cortical blood flow ("patchy defects") and reduced prefrontal metabolism [57] in abstinent cocaine abusers [58, 59]. Work investigating the stress response system suggests sustained changes in the stress response system following the development of opiate or cocaine dependence [48, 49]. Taken together, these studies suggest that the neurochemical and possibly the neuroendocrine systems of abstinent but formerly drug dependent patients, are functioning irregularly and at a reduced level for a very long time.

A second explanation for the enduring pathology seen among drug dependent persons and their tendency to become re-addicted lies in the integration of the reward circuitry with the motivational, emotional and memory centres that are co-located within the limbic system. Connections among these "survival circuits" are apparently designed to give prominence and emotional significance to the normal biological events that usually precede arousal of those circuits (food, danger, sex). These circuits are also intimately involved in the control of emotion, motivation and "biologically significant memories" [50, 51]. Importantly, these interconnected regions allow the organism not only to experience the pleasure of rewards, but also to learn the signals for them and to respond in an anticipatory manner.

This pairing of a person (drug using friend), place (corner bar), thing (paycheck), or even an emotional state (anger, depression) with drug use, including the supernormal activation of the reward circuits, leads to rapid and entrenched learning or "conditioning" to the point where these cues or signals acquire some of the properties of the drug itself. Thus, previously drug dependent individuals who have been abstinent for even long periods of time, may encounter a person, place or thing that has been previously associated with their drug use, producing significant physiological reactions. In the case of cocaine, these reactions include palpitations and other signs of sympathetic arousal such as ear-ringing, chest-tightness, light-headedness, a cocaine "taste" in the back of the throat [55]. In the case of heroin, this reaction includes pilo-erection, stomach cramps, fever and withdrawal-like symptoms [60]. Importantly, and regardless of the particular drug, these responses are usually accompanied by a profound desire or craving for that drug [55, 60]. Ingrained through learning, the confluence of the physiological, emotional and craving symptoms combine to produce the "loss of control" that has been considered a hallmark of drug dependence [14]. For example, Childress, O'Brien and their colleagues have shown the profound neurostimulation effects of cues that had been previously associated with use of drugs – even among stably abstinent former users [61]. Using positron emission tomography (PET) they compared regional cerebral blood flow in limbic and control brain regions of 14 detoxified male cocaine users and 6 cocaine-naive controls during exposure to neutral videos and to videos of cocaine-related scenes. During the cocaine video, former cocaine dependent subjects experienced increased craving and showed a pattern of limbic (amygdala and anterior cingulate) increases and basal ganglia decreases in regional cerebral blood flow. This pattern did not occur in cocaine-naive controls, nor among cocaine dependent patients in response to the neutral video or even to a different drug video [55]. These findings indicate that even rather artificial video scenes of cocaine-related stimuli, presented in the sterile and remote context of a PET laboratory, produced excitation of brain reward regions that mimicked the effects of the drug itself.

It is likely that both the direct and sustained physiological changes produced by the drugs themselves and the acquired effects produced by conditioned cues are involved in the ultimate explanation of the continued vulnerability to relapse even among motivated, abstinent, former drug dependent individuals [48]. At the same time, there is much left to explain here. As Childress has noted [55], all individuals have reward circuitry and most people have had their reward circuitry associated with natural reinforcers such as food, sex, sleep, and even some drug or alcohol use. Why don't all people use natural rewards compulsively? What distinguishes the brain function of those who use alcohol and other drugs but do not become addicted, from those who use similar amounts or at similar frequencies but do become dependent? Considered in combination with the heritability data from twin studies discussed above and data on congenital preference for alcohol and other drugs in specially bred strains of rats and mice it may be that alcohol, nicotine and other drugs have especially excitatory effects on particular "types" of individuals – or that the excitation of this circuitry is simply a parametric function of amount, duration, interval and frequency of drug administration – or both. These answers are not clear at this time and much more work needs to be done to identify the learned and innate aspects of vulnerability to drugs.

■ Part II. Are there effective medical treatments for addiction?

Regardless of whether the aetiology and course of addictive disorders are similar to those seen in other chronic diseases – the question of most import is whether these supposed diseases will actually *respond* to medications and other forms of medical treatment. To address this, we review the efficacy and effectiveness of treatment approaches for drug dependence compared against the untreated course of drug dependence; and, continuing our comparison with other forms of chronic medical illness, we consider whether and in what ways, the effectiveness of drug dependence treatment compares with the effectiveness of treatments for other chronic diseases such as hypertension, asthma and diabetes.

Standards for evaluating the effectiveness of drug dependence treatments

For the patient and particularly for the many treatment stakeholders in society, "effectiveness" of any medical treatment will be measured only in part by that treatment's initial effects on the presenting or primary symptoms. In fact, most treatments – especially those for chronic conditions and public health problems – are also evaluated in terms of their extended effects on the "disease related" problems that have limited personal function in the patient, that may have been costly to the health care system and/or may have become a public health concern to society [62]. These considerations also apply in the evaluation of treatments for addictive disorders. Typically, the immediate goal of reducing alcohol and drug use is necessary, but rarely sufficient, for the achievement of the longer term goals of improved personal health and social function. Thus, from the both patient's and society's perspectives, a truly "effective" treatment is one that not only provides lasting reduction of substance use, but also significantly improves personal and social functioning, particularly in areas of special public health and public safety concern. Again, these broad and diverse expectations of treatment are not peculiar to the addiction field. To quote Stewart and Ware in their recent text on outcome evaluation in general medical care [62]:

"... Since the 1970s however, the emphasis in America on what patient outcomes to measure to determine health status has been shifting... to the assessment of functioning, or the ability of the patients to perform the daily activities of their lives, how they feel, and their own personal evaluation of their health in general" [Ref. 62, p. 157].

Given that these issues are important in the treatment of drug dependence, not only to patients but also to society; addiction treatment outcomes have been measured on at least three domains [63]:

- Reduction of alcohol and drug use. The foremost goal of drug dependence treatments, measured objectively by urinalysis for drug screening and breathalyzer readings of blood alcohol content.
- Improvement in personal health, and social function: measures such as general health status inventories, psychological symptom inventories, family function measures and simple measures of days worked and dollars earned can be reliably and validly collected directly from the patient via confidential self report and/or from medical/psychiatric evaluations and employment records.
- Reduction in public health and public safety threats: threats to public health come from behaviors that spread infectious diseases and can be measured using standard laboratory tests for AIDS, STD's, TB and hepatitis. The commission of personal and property crimes can also be measured from public arrest and conviction records although these measures typically underestimate the extent of the criminal and dangerous behaviors actually performed [64].

In our view, the first two domains are quite consistent with the "primary and secondary measures of effectiveness" typically used by the Food and Drug Administration to evaluate new drug or device applications in controlled clinical trials [65] and as indicated above, quite consistent with the mainstream of thought regarding the evaluation of other forms of health care [63]. The final outcome dimension we believe is more specific to the treatment of drug dependence since it acknowledges the significant public health and public safety concerns associated with drug addiction. In the text that follows, we use these three domains to evaluate the published reports of drug dependence treatments with special emphasis upon medically oriented treatments.

Do treated Patients Show Better Outcomes Than Untreated Patients?

While it is not ethically possible to deny available treatment to those whose condition appears to require it, there are situations where treatments have not been applied to substance dependent persons and these situations offer some indication of what happens to substance use, personal function and the public health and safety problems of addicted individuals in the absence of treatment. Four recent studies provide information pertinent to this question.

Intravenous Drug Users

Metzger et al. [66] have examined the drug use, needle sharing practise and HIV infection rates of two large samples of opiate addicted patients in the Philadelphia area. Earlier studies of untreated intravenous drug users had shown reductions in drug injection rates and in needle sharing rates even from HIV testing alone [67-69]. However, in all of these studies, one third to one half of intravenous drug users showed no reductions in behaviors known to increase risk for the spread of infectious disease. Thus Metzger et al. [66] attempted to assess the effects of a medically oriented treatment for opiate dependence (methadone) in reducing HIV risk behaviors and the actual rates of HIV infection in two groups of heroin dependent individuals. The "In-Treatment" group was comprised of 152 patients randomly selected at admission to a large methadone maintenance program. These In-Treatment subjects were asked to refer their heroin using friends from the same neighborhoods who had been out of all substance dependence treatments for *at least one year*. This resulted in a group of 103 "Out of Treatment" heroin dependent individuals who were matched on age, race, gender, neighborhood and many other relevant background and social factors that are associated with drug use.

Both groups of patients were interviewed and tested for HIV status (90% contact rates at each interview) every six months over the next six years. Seropositive rates are displayed for both groups in *table I* above. As can be seen, at the initial assessment point, 13% of the In-Treatment sample and 21% of the Out-of-Treatment sample tested positive for HIV infection. By the six year point 51% of the Out-of-Treatment group, but only 21% of the In-Treatment group tested HIV positive [66]. It is important to note that without the untreated comparison group, data from the methadone group might have lead to a conclusion that treatment "did not work". That is, drug use had not been reduced to zero and there was still needle sharing in the treated group, but these risky behaviors were far less prevalent and less severe than seen among the matched group of untreated individuals.

Though the difference between the groups was quite remarkable, these data do not prove that treatment was the causal agent responsible for the different infection rates. It is possible and even likely, that the "out of treatment" subjects may have lacked the motivation for treatment found among the treated subjects, and this lack of desire for personal change, rather than the effects of the treatment itself, may have produced the status differences seen. For this reason, it is necessary to equate level of motivation, at least at the start of treatment, in order to make any valid judgment regarding the effectiveness of drug dependence treatment.

Waiting List Patients

An ongoing study of male veterans who applied for cocaine abuse treatment at the Philadelphia VA Medical Center helps to shed light on the relative outcomes of treated *vs* untreated patients who were approximately equal in their initial motivation for treatment. In this four-week study of waiting list patients by Urschel and his colleagues [70], sixty-eight cocaine dependent individuals

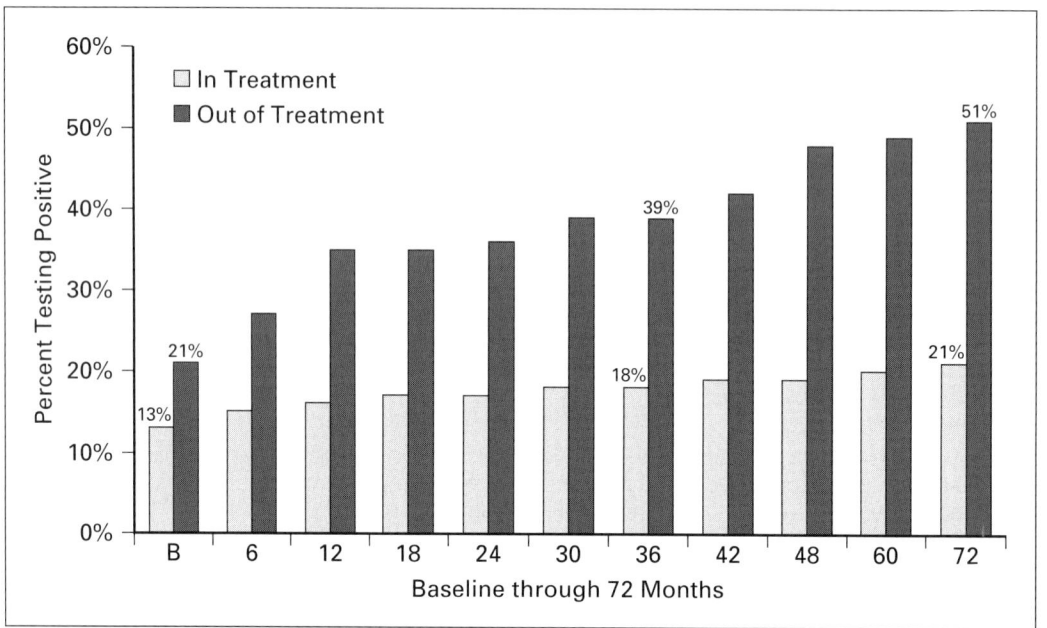

Table I. HIV Infection Rates Over Time.

were contacted at the time of their application for inpatient substance abuse treatment. Due to the unavailability of treatment beds, these individuals were put on a waiting list for treatment. These individuals were followed each week of their waiting period and asked questions regarding their drug use and health status, by independent evaluators. The question of interest was whether the cocaine use and the related problems would change without treatment in this group of individuals who were all at least initially motivated to change.

Results indicated that over the following four weeks only 16% of the group received any treatment related services (typically detoxification and/or temporary housing at a community shelter), and this small subgroup did show some reductions in their alcohol and other drug use, but no improvements in their health and social function. Among those who received no treatment services at all, 57% reported *increased* severity of medical problems and 81% reported *worse* employment and support problems over the four-week waiting period. Thus, there was little evidence from these data that the drug use or the related health problems showed significant improvement without treatment, despite the fact that they were clearly motivated for change.

Unmotivated individuals

Another way to separate the effectiveness of drug dependence treatment from the direct effects of motivation would be to compare treated and untreated substance dependent individuals who were *not* initially interested in treatment. Such a study was recently performed by Booth and associates [71] among intravenous drug users seeking HIV testing and AIDS services as part of a multi-site AIDS initiative involving 4,000 subjects recruited from fifteen cities. In each city that participated in the study, out-of-treatment injection drug users were offered an opportunity to participate in drug abuse treatment as a part of AIDS risk reduction services. In all cities, subjects were randomly assigned to either a "standard" HIV counselling and testing intervention or to an "enhanced" intervention consisting of the standard intervention plus one to three sessions of motivational counselling from a health educator. At six-month follow-up, those who were randomly assigned to the enhanced intervention showed half the rates of drug injection (20% *vs*

45%); four times the rates of abstinence (confirmed by urinalysis) and significantly lower arrest rates (14% vs 24%) than those randomly assigned to receive just HIV counselling and testing [71].

This study is significant for several reasons. First, the very modest public health efforts to reduce needle sharing and drug use through HIV counselling and testing were associated with significant reductions in these target behaviors – even among those who were not initially motivated to receive these interventions. Second, more extended but still modest efforts at referring patients into more formal treatment at seven of the study sites, were associated with broader and more sustained improvements not only in the target problems but in other areas such as abstinence, needle sharing and arrests. In turn, this finding suggests that treatment entry is not simply a matter of preconceived desire for change that would have occurred anyway – or the rates of treatment entry among these randomly assigned groups would have been approximately equal. Studies of other diseases show that even brief advice from physicians and other health care workers can affect the "motivation for treatment" among patients and the longer term course of their health [72, 73]. This is the very foundation of "primary care medicine" and as Booth et al. suggest, this also pertains even for seriously and chronically addicted individuals [71]. Appointments for a health care service of any type may set the occasion for brief screening and health counselling that can have important and lasting benefits not only for the addicted patient, but also for the broader public health.

The costs of untreated addiction: an example from prenatal care

A final study comparing the effects of drug abuse treatment to no treatment was performed by Svikis et al. [74] among one of the most problematic and costly subgroups of substance dependent individuals – pregnant women. The dangers of drug use during pregnancy are extreme both for the mother and the child [75-77]. Moreover, the costs associated with even the acute care of neonates born to addicted women can be extreme [78]. Thus the Svikis et al. study was designed to test the effects of standard drug dependence treatment *combined with* a standard program of prenatal and peri-natal care, on the health status and costs of the mothers and their children. As in the Booth et al. study, the effects of drug abuse treatment were assessed among individuals who did *not* originally apply for treatment. All subjects in the study had simply applied for prenatal care services and were found to be cocaine-positive on a routine drug screen. Two groups of pregnant women were compared: the first 100 women admitted to the combined drug dependence treatment-plus-pre-natal care program; and 46 comparison women drawn from the same geographic catchment area and matched for race, mental status, insurance coverage and parity with the treated women – but who were identified during the year prior to the opening of the experimental treatment program. Drug dependence treatment consisted of one week of non-hospital, residential care focused on stabilizing the women and engendering commitment for continued treatment, delivered in the context of their prenatal care. This was followed by twice-weekly addiction counselling that was also coordinated with the scheduled prenatal care visits.

Results were quite striking and three of the major findings are presented in *table II* above. With regard to the primary measure of drug use, 37% *of the treated patients had evidence of drug use (urinalysis) at the time of child birth*. Again, considered in the absence of a comparison group these data could lead to the conclusion that the treatment had failed. However, 63% *of the untreated women had cocaine positive urine tests at delivery*. The treated women kept twice the number of appointments as the untreated women (8 vs 4); the average birthweight was higher (2934 gms. vs 2539 gms.); and the gestational age of the baby was over one month higher at delivery (39 wks. vs 34 wks.). Following the deliveries, 10% of the babies in the treated group required treatment in the neonatal intensive care unit at an average length of stay of 7 days; as compared with 26% of the babies in the untreated group at an average length of stay of 39 days. The total costs of care for the mother and the baby in the treated group averaged approximately $14,500, including the costs for the drug abuse treatment. This was dramatically lower than the average costs of over $46,700 for the women and babies in the group that received prenatal care but no treatment for drug dependence. The authors point out that these average cost calculations were quite conservative since they did not include costs such as criminal and family court costs, child and family

Table II. Weight, Gestational Age & Costs.

46 Control Women	100 Treated Women
2,534 gms	*2,939 gms
34 wks	*39 wks
$46,700	$14,500

services, continued health care costs for mother and child, etc. Nonetheless, the data present striking evidence that drug dependence treatment can be cost effective in this severely affected population. The data also suggest that drug dependence treatment can be combined effectively with traditional perinatal medical care with mutual benefit.

Are drug dependence disorders responsive to medications?

If physicians are expected to play a role in the treatment of drug dependence, it is reasonable to ask whether there are effective medications available. Perhaps the best known and studied of medications in the treatment of drug dependence are those used in the treatment of smoking cessation such as nicotine gum, nicotine skin patch and buprorion (Zyban®). All of these medications were developed under FDA guidelines, researched in randomized clinical trials over the past twenty years and many have now reached the over-the-counter market. There is no doubt that these medications plus an educated physician population have made an important contribution in the larger public health efforts to reduce cigarette consumption.

A review of the evidence regarding the development of medications for the treatment of alcohol, cocaine and opiate addiction suggests many commonalities [40-43, 79, 80]. These medications have also been developing in the same manner – albeit more slowly due in part to the lack of a large commercial market – but the identification, development, testing of new drugs concurrent with necessary physician education practise have been major efforts in both the National Institutes on addictive disorders (NIDA, NIAAA) for the past five years [43]. These efforts have brought several existing medications to federal and state approval (*e.g.* LAAM, buprenorphine), identified important new uses for existing medications (*e.g.* naltrexone in alcohol treatment), and developed some promising new medications (*e.g.* buprenorphine, acamprosate). At the same time, there has been frustration in the development of an effective medication for cocaine addiction. Below, we review briefly several of the most prominent medications now available and some of the work in progress.

Medications for the Treatment of Opioid Addiction

Agonists, partial agonists and antagonists are the three primary types of medications available for the treatment of opioid dependence, all acting directly upon the opiate receptors – particularly mu-receptors [43]. Agonist medications are prescribed acutely as part of an opioid detoxification protocol (gradually reducing doses to minimize discomfort as the patient becomes acclimated to lower and finally zero doses of opiate); or chronically in a "maintenance" regimen (gradually increasing doses of long acting, pharmaceutical opiates to maximize the patient's tolerance and reduce or eliminate the effects of lower potency "street" opiates). Methadone has been an approved agonist medication for both the acute detoxification and the long term maintenance treatment of opiate dependence for more than 25 years. The long acting form of methadone (48-72 hour duration), Levo Alpha Acetyl Methadol (LAAM) has recently received FDA approval and has been accepted by 16 states for prescription – but only at methadone maintenance programs [81]. Double blind, placebo controlled trials have shown methadone to be effective in detoxifying opiate dependent patients safely and comfortably in both inpatient and outpatient settings [82-85]. As a maintenance medication, methadone's oral route of administration, slow onset of action and long half life have been very effective in reducing opiate use, crime and the spread of infectious diseases through needle sharing (*e.g.* AIDS, hepatitis, tuberculosis) for the past three decades. Recently, the effectiveness of methadone was supported by a National Institutes of Health consensus conference where evidence for methadone's effectiveness was reaffirmed by a panel of impartial physicians and scientists [86].

Partial agonist medications such as buprenorphine have also been developed over the past several years and have been widely used in Europe [87]. Buprenorphine is administered sub-lingually and has an effective duration of action of approximately 24-36 hours. Like methadone, buprenorphine significantly reduces craving for opiates and is currently being reviewed by the FDA. Large scale, double-blind, placebo controlled trials with buprenorphine have shown reductions in opiate use that are comparable to those seen with methadone [88]. The partial agonist actions of buprenorphine may have some advantages over methadone since it produces few or no withdrawal symptoms upon discontinuation of its use [87].

Opioid receptor antagonists such as naltrexone have also been used for more than 20 years in the treatment of opiate dependence [89]. Naltrexone is an orally administered opiate antagonist that blocks actions of externally administered opiates such as heroin through competitive binding for 48 to 72 hours [90-92]. Like methadone and buprenorphine naltrexone is a maintenance medication, designed as an "insurance policy" in situations where the patient is expected to be confronted with relapse situations. Opiate antagonists produce neither euphoria nor dysphoria when prescribed to abstinent opiate addicts, but as is true with so many maintenance medications in all other areas of medicine, compliance has been generally poor with most field studies showing retention rates of less than 20% after one month of treatment. Perhaps for this reason, several studies have combined this antagonist medication with social or criminal justice sanctions to increase compliance and sustain the benefits from the medication. For example, naltrexone is routinely used in the monitored treatment of physicians, lawyers, nurses and other professionals [93] where the loss of license to practise is contingent upon maintenance of abstinence. In a recent controlled trial with opiate dependent federal probationers Cornish *et al.* showed that naltrexone added to standard probation produced 70% less opiate use and 50% less re-incarceration rates than standard probation alone [94]. Like the Svikis study with pregnant cocaine dependent women, the Cornish study also showed that drug dependence treatments could be combined with other medical or social interventions with the potential for great cost savings [94].

Antagonist Medications in the treatment of Alcohol Dependence – Naltrexone (marketed under the trade name – Revia®)

It has been found to be effective in the treatment of alcohol dependence [95, 96] Naltrexone at 50 mg./day has been approved by the FDA for use with alcohol dependent patients since independent studies have shown it to be a safe, effective pharmacological adjunct for reducing heavy alcohol use among alcohol dependent patients. Its mechanism of action appears to be the blocking of at least some of the "high" produced by alcohol through competitive binding with mu opiate receptors [95, 96].

More recently, European researchers have found encouraging results using acamprosate to block craving and return to alcohol abuse. While acamprosate acts on different receptor systems than naltrexone, the clinical results are remarkably similar [97]. Alcohol dependent patients who take acamprosate have shown 30% greater post-treatment abstinence rates at six month follow-up than those randomly assigned to placebo. Further, those who have returned to drinking while receiving acamprosate report less heavy (greater than five drinks per day) alcohol use than those in the placebo group who returned to drinking [97]. While both of these medications can be used for extended periods, in practise they are generally prescribed for about one to three months as part of a more general rehabilitation program that includes behavioural change strategies [79].

Medications in the Treatment of Stimulant Dependence

Over the past ten years there have been many medications tried in the treatment of cocaine and other stimulant dependence. While this literature is quite large, it has been disappointing [for recent review see 80]. At this time of writing, there is no convincing evidence that any of the various types of cocaine blocking agents are truly effective for even brief periods of time or for even a significant minority of affected patients. Research continues in this important area and there have been indications of a potentially successful "vaccine" that may be able to immediately metabolize and inactivate active metabolites of cocaine [98]. This promising work is currently being tested in animal models and clinical trials will not be scheduled for several years. It must be admitted that at present there are no medications available that aid in cocaine rehabilitation.

Medications in the treatment of co-morbid psychiatric conditions

While we have briefly reviewed the still young literature on medications used to reduce or block the use of alcohol and other drugs, there is a large and important literature examining the use of medications to reduce psychiatric problems among addicted individuals [99-101]. This is an important area for physician involvement. Psychiatric disorders such as depression, anxiety, phobia and others are prominent among nicotine, alcohol, opiate, cocaine and benzodiazepine dependent individuals. There is abundant evidence that addicted individuals with concurrent psychiatric problems are more likely to drop out of standard drug dependence treatments, more likely to perform poorly during those treatments and more likely to relapse early following those treatments [102-104]. Finally, there is increasing evidence that the prescription of *appropriate* anti-depressant medications can alter that prognosis for these "psychiatrically more severe" individuals [99-101].

In summary, there are medications currently available for use by physicians in the treatment of nicotine, alcohol, and opioid dependence; and for the treatment of co-morbid psychiatric disorders associated with all forms of substance dependence. These have been tested in multiple trials and have been shown to be effective. At the same time there are still relatively few patients who receive – or practitioners who prescribe – these medications and, as in the treatment of other medical illnesses, managed care companies have been slow to authorize maintenance medications [42, 43, 80]. Because of this there is a need for additional studies of the appropriate use of these medications in "real world" treatment of drug dependence disorders.

Is drug dependence responsive to brief physician interventions?

One of the most interesting and potentially important developments over the past decade has been the research in physician administered brief interventions as part of office-based primary care [105-111]. These interventions follow the identification of "at risk" drinking or drug use through any number of simple screening instruments. Once the problem has been identified the physician begins a nonchallenging discourse with the patient designed to get the patient to accept that there is a problem and that the patient has the ability to correct the problem. Problem acceptance (*i.e.* that the patient is drinking too much) by a patient can be difficult but direct assessment of the problem and simple feedback of normal behaviors (*e.g.* simple charts showing normal levels of drinking by age and gender) can be much more helpful than scolding or confrontation [112]. Patient behavioural change is accomplished through negotiation of some behavioural goals that are agreed upon by contracting with patient [105-107]. These brief interventions (usually 10 to 20 minutes of physician time in the office) have typically been accompanied by brief booklets or self-help manuals and regular follow-up, usually over the phone. In many ways, these brief interventions for problematic alcohol and drug use are similar to the types of interventions used in the office-based, primary care management of other chronic illnesses.

Clinical research in office-based settings has shown these approaches to be both effective and cost saving [108-111]. For example, a study of office-based brief interventions by Kristenson in Sweden showed sustained reductions in alcohol use (verified by liver function tests) and healthcare utilization [108]. A second study performed by the Medical Research Council in England with 47 general practitioners found more significant reductions in alcohol use in the intervention group than in the randomly assigned control (no intervention) group, twelve months following the intervention [109]. A World Health Organization study of brief interventions in ten countries also studied brief interventions in both physician offices and in general clinic settings [110]. When the total sample was analyzed, there were approximately equal reductions in alcohol use among both the control group (who had simply had their alcohol use identified and reported to them) and the brief intervention group. However, when data from just the physician offices was analyzed there was a significant effect of the brief intervention. Brief interventions were also studied in 17 community physician office practise by Fleming *et al.* [111]. In that study "at risk drinkers" were screened and offered two, 10-15 minutes interventions by the physician, or simply provided a health booklet. Risk was defined as the self-reported drinking of more than 13 or 10 drinks in the past week for men and women, respectively. At both six and twelve month follow-up the intervention group was drinking on fewer days, drinking significantly less, reporting fewer binge drinking episodes (greater than 4 or 5 more drinks per occasion for women and men, respectively) and hospitalized for fewer days – than the control group. A follow-up study of costs and benefits [113] showed 5: 1 savings per dollar invested in the intervention. Most of the savings came from reduced hospital days and emergency room visits as well as avoided crime and motor vehicle accidents [113].

Several points are relevant here. First, these interventions do require training (about one and one-half hours for the physician and the same for an office nurse) [113]. The training is designed to help physicians avoid confrontation and to develop constructive methods of engaging the patient into the behavioural change that will be required. Second, these interventions require some form of screening for alcohol and drug problems, but there are many patient-administered screening instruments available. Third, while these interventions have been studied in the context of alcohol treatment, these behavioural change initiation skills would be broadly useful in the treatment of most other forms of chronic illness. Finally, while the results reported here have been broadly replicated, it is likely that these brief forms of intervention are more appropriate for, and accepted by individuals with lower levels of problem severity. Further, these brief interventions have not been studied in populations of drug abusers. It therefore remains a question whether these minimal types of interventions would be effective for patients with more serious alcohol and particularly, drug abuse problems.

Treatment adherence in drug dependence and other chronic diseases?

There is no reliable "cure" for drug dependence. For the reasons cited above, persons dependent upon nicotine, alcohol, opiates, cocaine, barbiturates or marijuana who attempt to reduce their use are likely to have problems in maintaining "controlled use". Among those who become addicted, studies of treatment response have uniformly shown that those patients who comply with the recommended regimen of education, counselling and medication that characterizes most contemporary forms of drug dependence treatment, have the most favourable outcomes during and following treatment [114-118]. Despite this, most of those who start any type of treatment drop out prior to completion and/or ignore advice to continue medications or aftercare or AA participation following formal treatment. Even those who do comply with treatment fully have problems sustaining abstinence, with one year follow-up studies indicating that only 40-60% of treated patients are able to remain completely abstinent throughout that time period, although an additional 15-30% do not resume dependent use or develop problems associated with drug use [118-120 also see below].

It is quite discouraging to many in the treatment field that so many drug and alcohol dependent patients fail to comply with the recommended course of treatment and that so many of those who complete treatment subsequently resume substance use. Recent reviews of the treatment literature have indicated that factors such as low socioeconomic class, co-morbid psychiatric conditions and lack of family or social supports for continuing abstinence are among the most important variables associated with lack of treatment compliance in this field, and with relapse following treatment [121]. As indicated above there are now several medications that have demonstrated effectiveness in the treatment of alcohol and opiate dependence. However, for these medications to be effective, they must be taken on a regular basis and lack of patient compliance has severely limited the potential impact of these medications [122]. Ongoing clinical research in this area is focused upon the development of longer acting or depot forms of these medications, as well as behavioural strategies to increase patient compliance [122].

As suggested previously, hypertension, diabetes and asthma are also chronic disorders, requiring continuing care for most, if not all of a patient's life. At the same time, these disorders are not necessarily unremitting or unalterably lethal, *as long as the treatment regimen of medication, diet and behavioural change are followed.* This last point requires emphasis. Treatments for these medical disorders are heavily dependent upon behavioural change and medication compliance to achieve their potential effectiveness. In a review of over 70 outcome studies of treatments for these disorders patient compliance with the recommended medical regimen was the most significant determinant of treatment outcome [123, 124]. However, studies have shown that less than 50% of Type 2, insulin dependent, adult diabetics fully comply with their medication schedule [e.g. 125], and less than 30% of hypertensive or asthmatic patients comply with their medication regimens [e.g. 126, 127]. The problem is even worse for the behavioural and diet changes that are so important for the maintenance of short term gains in these chronic disorders. Again, a review of recent studies in the fields of adult onset diabetes, hypertension and asthma indicates that less than 30% of patients in treatment for these disorders comply with the recommended diet and/or behavioural changes that are designed to reduce risk factors for reoccurence of the disorders [e. g. 128, 129]. Across all three of these chronic medical illnesses, compliance is poorest among patients with low socioeconomic status, low family and social supports or significant psychiatric co-morbidity as is summarized in table III below.

Table III. Factors associated with relapse in hypertension, diabetes & asthma.

#1	Lack of adherence to medication, diet, or behavior change
#2	Low socioeconomic status
#3	Low family supports
#4	Psychiatric co-morbidity

Sources: National Center Health Stats; Harrison, 13th Ed. (more than 30 published studies).

Relapse rate in drug dependence and other chronic diseases?

This review of medication and behavioural compliance in the treatment of other chronic medical illnesses suggests important parallels with the treatment of drug dependence. As in the field of drug dependence treatment, lack of patient compliance with the treatment regimen is a major contributor to the reoccurence of these disorders and to the development of more serious and more expensive "disease related" conditions. For example, outcome studies indicate that 30-60% of insulin dependent, adult, diabetic patients, and approximately 50-80% of adult hypertensive and asthmatic patients suffer reoccurences of their symptoms each year to the point that they require at least, restabilization of their medication and/or additional medical interventions to re-establish symptom remission [125-129]. Many of these recurrences also result in more serious additional health complications. For example, limb amputations and blindness are common results of treatment non response among diabetics [130, 131]. Stroke and cardiac disease are common problems associated with exacerbation of hypertension [132, 133]. These recurrence or relapse rates are summarized in table IV below.

Table IV. Relapse* Rates for Chronic Medical Disorders.

Hypertension	50-60%
Diabetes	30-50%
Asthma	60-80%

* Relapse = Retreated w/in 12 months, in ER or Hospital.

■ Part III. What are the "active ingredients" in addiction treatment?
What components contribute to treatment effectiveness?

The detoxification-stabilization phase of treatment

Medical detoxification has been the initial and acute stage of virtually all forms of addiction treatment. However, the term "detoxification" has been used to describe both treatments of a true withdrawal syndrome (i.e., neuroadaptation) as well as simply the stabilization of acute physiological and emotional symptoms associated with the cessation of drug use that might not produce a bona fide withdrawal syndrome. "True detoxification" is required only for certain types of drug dependence, most notably nicotine, alcohol, opiate, barbiturate, and benzodiazepines. In each of these cases (particularly barbiturate use) persistent use of a substance at gradually escalating doses and for escalating time periods produces neuroadaptation or "tolerance" to the drug – to the point where greater amounts of the drug are typically required to produce euphoria – and importantly – eliminate withdrawal symptoms. Withdrawal symptoms reflect the "rebound" of a physiological system that has been perturbed by drug use for a substantial period of time. These symptoms can include headaches, bone pain, fever, chills, watery eyes, runny nose, diarrhea and profound emotional upset. Opiate drugs in particular can produce these symptoms and while they are profoundly uncomfortable, they are rarely life threatening. Importantly, alcohol, barbiturates and benzodiazepines will also produce many of the previously described symptoms – but also seizures and cardiac irregularities – that can be life threatening depending upon the history and general health of the user.

It is also true that virtually all drug use – including caffeine, amphetamine, cocaine and hallucinogens – will produce acute periods (1-3 days typically) of physiological and emotional instability following abrupt discontinuation of regular use. While uncomfortable, this instability will almost always subside without formal medical attention. Thus, at least in the United States, few patients are admitted to a hospital or even to residential care for the acute treatment of the instability produced by these drugs. Although cocaine "withdrawal" has been recognized in the *Diagnostic and Statistical Manual*, Fourth Edition (*DSM IV*, see 14], there is continued debate regarding the treatment and even the existence of a bona fide withdrawal syndrome following cocaine use [134, 135]. At the same time, there is clear agreement that patients who have used cocaine or crack continuously over sustained periods, suffer two to five day periods of measurable physiological and psychiatric instability [136, 137]. For this reason, cocaine "stabilization" is included in this review along with formal detoxification.

Goals of Detoxification-Stabilization

- *Patients and treatment settings.* The detoxification and stabilization phase of treatment is designed for patients who have been actively abusing alcohol or street drugs, or both, and who are suffering physiological or emotional instability, or both. In cases of severe withdrawal potential or extreme physiological or emotional instability, detoxification-stabilization helps to prevent serious medical consequences of abrupt withdrawal, to reduce the physiological and emotional signs of instability, and to motivate necessary behavioural change strategies that will be the focus of rehabilitation. This stage of treatment may take place in inpatient settings, either a hospital or a non-hospital, residential setting, or in outpatient settings, such as in a hospital-based clinic or a residential or social setting.

- *Treatment Elements and Methods.* Medications are available for both physiological withdrawal signs and for the temporary relief of acute medical problems associated with physiological instability (*e.g.*, sleep medications, antidiarrheal medications, vitamins, and nutritional supplements). Motivational counselling is widely used to address shame and ambivalence, as well as to increase adherence with recommendations for continued rehabilitation.

- *Duration.* Regardless of the setting, stabilization of acute problems is typically completed within 2 to 10 days, with the average being 3 to 5 days [138]. True detoxification is necessary only for cases of severe alcohol, opiate, benzodiazepine, or barbiturate use, although many cocaine-dependent and other drug-dependent patients suffer from significant physiological and emotional instability that precludes immediate participation in rehabilitation. The duration of the detoxification-stabilization process depends on the presence and severity of the patient's dependence symptoms as well as concurrent medical and psychiatric problems. Treatments longer than 5 days are unusual and typically are due to conjoint medical or psychiatric problems or physiological dependence upon some forms of sedatives (*e.g.*, alprazolam).

Effective Components of the Detoxification-Stabilization Stage of Treatment

- *Setting of Care: Medical or Nonmedical and Inpatient or Outpatient.* Debate regarding the appropriate setting of care in which to detoxify alcohol-dependent patients has been substantial.

Since the mid-1970s, medical settings such as residential treatment facilities or even outpatient treatment centres have conducted detoxification or stabilization treatments for alcohol, opiates, and more recently, cocaine. Although studies have not systematically compared social settings with medical settings for detoxification from alcohol dependence, there are reports of favourable outcomes in both.

In the presence of significant physiological signs of alcohol, opiate, benzodiazepine, or barbiturate withdrawal however, the standard treatment includes medical supervision in either a hospital or an outpatient medical clinic [138]. Although research is not extensive, medical settings are generally viewed as being more appropriate for detoxifications involving medical problems (particularly those with a history of seizures) and psychiatric problems (particularly for individuals with depression and at risk of suicide) and also when patients have concurrent cocaine dependence.

- *Alcohol Detoxification.* Within the framework of medically supervised alcohol detoxification, the relative effectiveness and costs of inpatient *versus* outpatient alcohol detoxification have been examined [139, 140]. In a study by Hayashida *et al.* [139], chronic alcohol-dependent patients without histories of serious psychiatric or medical complications were randomly assigned to receive medically supervised alcohol withdrawal in either an inpatient or a day-hospital setting. On two of the outcome domains considered important for detoxification treatments (safe elimination of withdrawal signs and engagement in ongoing rehabilitation), the inpatient group showed significantly better performance, but the re-addiction rates were less than 12% for both groups. Despite this statistically significant advantage for the inpatient setting, it was 10 times more costly than outpatient detoxification in an outpatient setting.

  There may be some advantage to inpatient detoxification when a patient does not have the social or personal supports necessary to comply with the outpatient attendance requirements. However, despite somewhat lower retention rates for outpatient than for inpatient alcohol detoxification [139, 140], outpatient detoxification may be more acceptable to a wider range of drinkers who wish to avoid the stigma of treatment in a designated detoxification unit [140].

- *Opiate Detoxification.* Available evidence suggests that opiate detoxification can be accomplished with many medications including clonidine, lofexidine, buprenorphine and of course methadone. Recently there have been reports of rapid (24 hours or less) opiate detoxification under general sedation [141]. There are at least four reports in the literature showing the "efficacy" of this method, but there are also some elevated dangers associated with this modality as applied in general practise [142]. Apart from these relatively new procedures, a wealth of studies over the past ten years have shown that opiate detoxifications can generally be accomplished in outpatient settings under medical supervision with gradually reduced doses of methadone [143, 144]. However, completion rates for treatment of opioid dependence may be higher in inpatient than in outpatient detoxification programs [145, 146].

- *Cocaine, Crack and Other Stimulant Stabilization.* Few studies have examined the appropriate setting for the stabilization of physiological and psychiatric signs and symptoms associated with extended cocaine or crack use. The prevailing practise has been to attempt to stabilize all but the most severely affected patients through outpatient care. Patients who are in the acute stages of cocaine cessation and who are more severely affected (medically or psychiatrically) are placed into a hospital if they have significant cardiac problems or significant psychiatric symptomatology or are at least placed in inpatient social settings for the first 3 to 5 days of cocaine treatment [136-138].

The available literature is replete with accounts of early dropouts during the first 2 to 3 weeks of outpatient cocaine treatment [147-149], with attrition rates ranging from a low of 27% to a high of 47% in the first few weeks of care. As discussed below, it is reasonable to conclude that the patients with the most severe medical and psychiatric problems are most susceptible to drop out of treatment early.

Length of Stay and Criteria for Completion

Alcohol and Opiates

Several detoxification studies [139, 143] have measured detoxification as 3 consecutive days of abstinence from observable withdrawal signs or symptoms (opiate or alcohol), using standardized inventories of these physical measures. Using these criteria, the great majority of detoxifications can be accomplished in 3 to 5 days [138], and there is no evidence of greater effectiveness from extended stays.

In an early study by Cushman et al. [143], only 3% of 525 opiate-dependent patients who failed to provide an opiate-negative urine specimen following the outpatient detoxification (signifying at least 3 days of abstinence) were able to engage in the suggested abstinence-oriented rehabilitation program following detoxification. One hundred percent of these patients were re-addicted to opiates at the 6-month follow-up.

Cocaine

A recent study of cocaine-dependent patients entering outpatient rehabilitation also offers some relevant information on the clinical importance of developing a criterion for successful completion. In a study of cocaine-dependent veterans, Alterman et al. [147] found that the single best predictor of engagement into the rehabilitation process, and ultimately program completion (elimination of cocaine use verified by urinalysis), was the presence or absence of cocaine metabolites in the urine sample submitted upon admission to the rehabilitation program, signifying recent cocaine use. Of those patients without cocaine metabolites present in their urine on admission, 79% engaged in and completed the outpatient treatment, whereas only 39% of those with a positive urine sample on admission engaged and completed the outpatient treatment.

Indicators of Effectiveness in the Detoxification-Stabilization Stage

The therapeutic goals of detoxification and stabilization are focused primarily on the amelioration and stabilization of the acute medical, psychiatric, or substance use symptoms that were out of control and thus responsible for preventing the patient from entering directly into rehabilitation. Thus, the goal of detoxification-stabilization is removal of the physiological and emotional instability that has impeded direct entry to rehabilitative treatment – as well as motivating the patient to recognize the severity of the drug use, to accept that there is a problem that s/he must and can address, and to engage the patient in continued rehabilitative care, almost always in an outpatient setting. The acute, detoxification/stabilization stage *cannot* be considered complete treatment – only *preparation* for continued treatment. Research over the past 20 years in most countries has concluded definitively that detoxification is associated with lasting improvements *only* when there is continued rehabilitative treatment [1]. Thus, detoxification can be said to have succeeded if shortly after discharge (*i.e.*, 2-3 weeks) the patient has:

– shown significant reductions in physiological and emotional instability (at least to levels appropriate for outpatient rehabilitation admission),
– has not had serious medical or psychiatric complications,
– and has been integrated into and engaged in an appropriate ongoing rehabilitation program.

The rehabilitation-relapse prevention phase of treatment

Patients and Treatment Settings

Rehabilitation is appropriate for patients who are no longer suffering from the acute physiological or emotional effects of recent substance use and who need behavioural change strategies to regain control of their urges to use substances. Rehabilitation may be initiated in a residential setting *but sustained benefits require that it continue beyond that setting* – since life in a controlled environment does not permit the patient to practise the skills necessary to prevent a relapse to substance use. Thus, most rehabilitation takes place in outpatient clinics or social settings. A practical goal of this stage of treatment is to prevent a return to active substance use that would require re-detoxification/stabilization; to assist the patient in developing control over urges to use alcohol or drugs, or both, usually through sustaining total abstinence from all drugs and alcohol; and to assist the patient in regaining or attaining improved personal health and social function, both as a secondary part of the rehabilitation function and because these improvements in lifestyle are important for maintaining sustained control over substance use.

Treatment elements and methods

Professional opinions vary widely regarding the underlying reasons for the loss of control over alcohol and/or drug use typically seen in treated patients. For example, genetic predispositions, acquired metabolic abnormalities, learned, negative behavioural patterns, deeply ingrained feelings of low self-worth, self-medication of underlying psychiatric or physical medical problems, character flaws, and lack of family and community support for positive function have all been suggested as mechanisms. Thus, there is an equally wide range of treatment strategies and treatments that can be used to correct or ameliorate these underlying problems and to provide continuing support for the targeted patient changes.

Strategies have included such diverse elements as psychotropic medications to relieve "underlying psychiatric problems"; medications to relieve alcohol and drug cravings; acupuncture to correct acquired metabolic imbalances; educational seminars, films, and group sessions to correct false impressions about alcohol and drug use; group and individual counselling and therapy sessions to provide insight, guidance, and support for behavioural changes; and peer help groups (*e.g.*, Alcoholics Anonymous [AA] and Narcotics Anonymous [NA]) to provide continued support for the behavioural changes thought to be important for sustaining improvement.

Duration

Typically, residential rehabilitation treatments range from 30 to 90 days; outpatient, abstinence-oriented forms of treatment range from 30 to 120 days; therapeutic community modalities typically range from 6 months to 1 year; and methadone maintenance can have an indefinite time period.

Many of the more intensive forms of outpatient treatment (intensive outpatient and day hospital) begin with full or half-day sessions five or more times per week for approximately 1 month. As the rehabilitation progresses, the intensity of the treatment reduces to shorter-duration sessions of 1 to 2 hours delivered twice per week and tapering to once per week. The final part of outpatient treatment is typically called "continuing care" or "aftercare", with biweekly to monthly group support meetings continuing (in association with parallel activities in self-help groups) for as long as 2 years.

Maintenance medications

Although the majority of rehabilitation treatment programs in the United States are abstinence-oriented, a significant number of rehabilitation programs maintain patients on a medication that is designed to block the effects of the abused drugs (*e.g.*, acamprosate, disulfiram or naltrexone to block alcohol abuse), thus preventing the re-emergence of drug use. In the case of opiates and nicotine, many patients are "maintained" on a medication that is designed to override the effects of the abused drugs in what may seem a paradoxical way – through the development of greater physiological tolerance to the same class of drugs. While more tolerance is typically developed during the course of medication with these maintenance drugs, the tolerance is to a safer, more potent, and longer-acting medication from within the class of abused drugs. For example, nicotine patch provides significant doses of nicotine, elevating tolerance to nicotine but preventing withdrawal that abstinence would induce and obviating the need for cigarettes to provide the nicotine. In the same way, methadone, LAAM and buprenorphine produce more opioid tolerance in an opioid abuser – but again, no worries about withdrawal and no need for heroin.

Maintenance forms of treatment are always controversial since many in the public and even those in the treatment field believe that medications are just another form of "drug", and that all drug usage should be eliminated. However, if one takes a broader, medical perspective on this form of rehabilitative care, these medication maintenance approaches are quite similar to current strategies for ameliorating the physiological or emotional problems in individuals with other chronic medical conditions, such as long-term maintenance on antidepressant, antipsychotic, or other psychotropic medications for psychiatric patients; maintenance on beta-blockers and other normotensive agents for patients with hypertension; antiasthmatics for asthma sufferers; and insulin for diabetics. A substantial amount of research has shown that these medications can be very effective in the rehabilitation of several forms of addiction [144, 150, 151].

Defining outcomes

All forms of rehabilitation oriented treatments for addiction have the same four goals, regardless of the specific setting, modality, philosophy, or methods of rehabilitation. These are to:

- maintain the physiological and emotional improvements that were initiated during detoxification-stabilization phase, preventing need for re-detoxification,
- enhance and sustain reductions in alcohol and drug use (most rehabilitation programs suggest a goal of complete abstinence),
- teach, model and encourage behaviors that lead to improved personal health, improved social function, and reduced threats to public health and public safety, and
- teach and motivate behavioural and lifestyle changes that are incompatible with substance abuse.

It is important to note the purposely broad perspective on measuring effectiveness as was discussed in Part 1. Specifically, for any form of substance abuse rehabilitation intervention to be worthwhile to society, *there must be lasting improvements in those problems that led to the treatment admission and that are important to the patient and to society*. This definition purposely emphasizes improvements that have an enduring or lasting quality [152-155]. Because these disorders are chronic and relapsing, a "cure" for substance use disorders is not now achievable in most cases. Nonetheless, there are many illnesses that cannot be cured and yet there are "effective treatments" for these illnesses that arrest and contain symptoms and permit improved function. The definition also emphasizes those improvements that are important to society. For the many parts of society affected by substance abuse, the effectiveness of treatment will be measured by the extended effects of treatment on the addiction-related problems that have become public health and public safety concerns. Given this framework, it can be seen that achievement of the primary goal of reducing alcohol and drug use is *necessary, but not always sufficient*, to improve the addiction-related problems that are typically so prominent among individuals seeking treatment. Furthermore, without additional improvements in these associated problems, addiction treatment may not be worthwhile *either* to the patient who undergoes it or to the society that supports it [152-155].

Effective components in the rehabilitation – relapse prevention stage of treatment

Using the above framework for defining outcome, we now summarize briefly, some of the many studies that have investigated treatment processes and treatment components in order to determine the "active ingredients" of the rehabilitation stage of treatment, and who appears to benefit most from these ingredients. Until only recently patient factors had been more thoroughly studied than treatment process factors with regard to their role in treatment outcome. With the development of new medications and behavioural interventions there are now many studies devoted to the exploration of treatment "ingredients" or elements and their role in post-treatment outcome. Below, we review several of the more prominent factors.

Medications

Great progress has been made over the past ten years in the development of new medications and in the application of existing medications for the treatment of particular conditions associated with substance dependence and for particular types of substance dependent patients. This progress has been summarized above in Part II.

Setting of Treatment

There have now been many studies investigating differences in outcome between various forms of inpatient and outpatient rehabilitation. For example, studies by McCrady et al. [156] and Alterman et al. [157] randomly assigned alcohol dependent patients to an equal length (28-30 days) of either inpatient or day-hospital rehabilitation, where the treatment elements were also designed to be similar. Both studies showed very similar findings. Patients in both the inpatient and outpatient arms of both these studies showed substantial and significant reductions in alcohol use, as well as improvements in many other areas of personal health and social function – suggesting that both settings of care were able to produce substantial benefits. At the same time, a wide range of outcome measures collected at six month follow-up in both studies, showed essentially no statistically significant or clinically important differences between the two settings of care – suggesting that the setting of care might not be an important contributor to outcome.

Other reviews of the literature on inpatient and outpatient alcohol rehabilitation by Miller and Hester [158] and Holder et al. [159], also concluded that across a range of study designs and patient populations there are few significant advantages provided by inpatient care over outpatient care in the rehabilitation of alcohol dependence, despite the substantial difference in costs. In contrast, a widely cited study by Walsh et al. [160] did find a significant difference in outcome favouring an inpatient program. However, this difference was shown among employed alcohol dependent patients who were assigned to either an inpatient program plus Alcoholics Anonymous (AA) or to AA meetings only (rather than to formal outpatient treatment). One recent review of the alcohol inpatient-outpatient literature did conclude that in studies that found an advantage to inpatient care over outpatient treatment, outpatients did not receive inpatient detoxification and the studies tended to not have social stability inclusion criteria or to require randomization [161]. This review points to the need to consider "real world" factors when evaluating the effectiveness of different treatment settings.

In the field of cocaine dependence treatment, there have also been several studies examining the role of treatment setting. Again, while there have typically been high attrition rates [e.g. 148], there is still evidence indicting that outpatient treatments for cocaine dependence can be effective, even for patients with relatively limited social resources. For example, Alterman and his colleagues followed up a prior comparison study of inpatient and day-hospital treatment of alcohol dependence [156] with an identical examination comparing the effectiveness of four weeks of intensive, highly structured day hospital treatment (27 hours weekly) with that of inpatient treatment (48 hours weekly) for cocaine dependence. The subjects were primarily inner city, male African Americans treated at a Veterans Administration Medical Center. The inpatient treatment completion rate of 89% was significantly higher than the day-hospital completion rate of 54%. However, at seven months post treatment entry, self reported outcomes indicated considerable improvements for both groups in drug and alcohol use, family/social, legal, employment, and psychiatric problems. The finding of reduced self reported cocaine use was supported by urine screening results. Both self report and urine data indicated 50-60% abstinence for both groups at the follow-up assessment. The comparability of both treatment settings was also evident in 12 month outcomes in both randomized and self-selecting patients [162].

There have been at least two attempts to formalize clinical decision processes regarding who should, and should not be assigned to inpatient and outpatient settings of care (Cleveland Criteria; American Association of Addiction Medicine Criteria). McKay et al. [97] failed to show evidence for the predictive validity of the Cleveland placement criteria at least when applied to the assignment of alcohol and drug dependent patients to day hospital or inpatient care. That is, patients who met the Cleveland criteria for inpatient treatment did not have worse outcomes than those who met criteria for day hospital only when both groups received day hospital treatment. If the Cleveland Criteria had been valid, those who "needed inpatient treatment" but did not receive it should have had poorer outcomes than those who were appropriately "matched" to day hospital. In a similar study evaluating the psychosocial predictors from the American Association of Addiction Medicine (ASAM) criteria, McKay et al. [163] did find at least partial support for the predictive validity of these placement variables. That is, among patients who "needed inpatient treatment" as defined by the *psychosocial elements* of the ASAM criteria, those who were randomly assigned to outpatient care did show somewhat worse abstinence rates and generally poorer social outcomes than those who were randomly assigned to inpatient rehabilitation. The retrospective nature of this study made it impossible to complete a full evaluation of these criteria.

The most recent versions of the ASAM criteria have attempted to make very fine grained decisions regarding placements to levels of care defined by the amount and quality of medical supervision and monitoring. Research is needed to determine the predictive validity of these finer distinctions and whether placements to settings and modalities with "more medical supervision" actually receive more medical contact or services than placements that are not expected to receive such services.

Length of treatment/compliance with treatment

Perhaps the most robust and pervasive indicator of favourable post treatment outcome in all forms of substance abuse rehabilitation has been length of stay in treatment. Virtually all studies of rehabilitation have shown that patients who stay in treatment longer and/or attend more treatment sessions, have better post treatment outcomes [164-168]. Specifically, several studies have suggested that outpatient treatments of less than 90 days are more likely to result in early return to drug use and generally poorer response than treatments of longer duration [164, 167, 168].

Though length of stay is a very robust, positive predictor of treatment outcome, the nature of this relationship is still ambiguous. Clearly, one possibility is that patients who enter treatment gradually acquire new motivation, skills, attitudes, knowledge, and supports over the course of their stay in treatment; that those who stay longer acquire more of these favourable attributes and qualities; and that the gradual acquisition of these qualities or services is the reason for the favourable outcomes. An equally plausible possibility is that "better motivated and better adjusted patients" come into treatment ready and able to change; that the decisions they made to "change their lives" were made in advance of their admission and because of this greater motivation and "treatment readiness" they are likely to stay longer in treatment and to do more of what is recommended. These two interpretations of the same facts have very different implications for treatment practise. If treatment gradually produces positive changes over time, it is obviously clinically sound practise to retain patients longer – perhaps even through coercion – and to provide them with more services during treatment. On the other hand, if well motivated, high functioning, compliant patients enter treatment with the requisite skills and supports necessary to do well, then efforts to provide more services or to coerce patients into longer stays may not add to the effectiveness of more streamlined and less expensive rehabilitation efforts.

Participation in AA/NA

AA is of course recognized as a self-help or mutual support organization and not a formal treatment. For this reason, and because of the anonymous quality of the group, much less research has been done to evaluate this important part of substance abuse rehabilitation [169, 170]. While there has always been consensual agreement on the value of AA and other peer support forms of treatment, new evidence has emerged over the past five years showing that patients who have an AA sponsor, or who have participated in the fellowship activities – have much better abstinence records than patients who have received rehabilitation treatments but have not continued in AA. McKay and his colleagues [171] found that participation in post treatment self-help groups predicted better outcome among a group of cocaine or alcohol dependent veterans in a day hospital rehabilitation program. Timko et al. [172], found that more AA attendance was associated with better 1-year outcomes among previously untreated problem drinkers regardless of whether they received inpatient, outpatient, or no other treatment. Finally, a recent review of the literature on the impact of self-help programs concluded that greater participation was generally associated with better alcohol and psychosocial outcomes, although the magnitude of the effects tended to vary as a function of the quality of the study and whether patients were treated in inpatient or outpatient settings [173].

There has been less research into the use of self-help organizations among cocaine and/or opiate dependent patients. However, a recent study of cocaine patients participating in outpatient counselling and psychotherapy showed that while only 34% attended a cocaine anonymous (CA) meeting, 55% of those who did became abstinent as compared with only 38% of those who did not attend CA.

It is difficult to sort out the extent to which AA attendance is an active ingredient of successful treatment and/or the extent to which it is simply a marker for general treatment compliance and commitment to abstinence. In this regard, several investigators have studied the relationship of completing various 12-step processes during the course of rehabilitation, to relapse following treatment. Morgenstern et al. reported that patients who adopted more of the attitudinal and behavioural tenets of the 12-step model of rehabilitation such as admission of powerlessness, acceptance of a higher power, commitment to AA, and agreement that alcoholism is a disease, were no more (or less) likely to relapse following treatment than patients who had adopted very few of the 12-step tenets by the end of the rehabilitation treatment [174]. At the same time, two general tenets found in all rehabilitation models – greater commitment to abstinence and greater intention to avoid high risk situations – did predict a lower likelihood of relapse [174]. In another analysis from the same study, greater affiliation with AA following treatment predicted better outcomes. AA affiliation was in turn positively associated with self-efficacy, motivation, and coping efforts, which were themselves significant predictors of outcome [174]. Thus, more research in this area is warranted to determine how participation in AA exerts its positive effects.

The therapist or counsellor

Research also suggests that having access to regular drug/alcohol counselling can make an important contribution to the engagement and participation of the patient in treatment and to the post treatment outcome. One example of the role of the counsellor and of individual counselling was shown in a study of methadone maintained patients, all within the same treatment program and all receiving the same methadone dose, who were randomly assigned to receive counselling or no counselling in addition to the methadone [175]. Results showed that 68% of patients assigned to the no counselling condition failed to reduce drug use (confirmed by urinalysis) and 34% of these patients required at least one episode of emergency medical care. In contrast, no patient in the counselling groups required emergency medical care, 63% showed sustained elimination of opiate use and 41% showed sustained elimination of cocaine use over the six months of the trial.

A study by Fiorentine [176] as part of a larger "Target Cities" evaluation also showed the contribution of counselling in drug rehabilitation. Group counselling was the most common modality (averaging 9.5 sessions per month) followed by 12-step meetings (average 7.5 times per month) and individual counselling (average 4.7 times per month). Greater frequency of both group and individual counselling sessions were shown to decrease the likelihood of relapse over the subsequent six months. One important contribution of this study, given the above cautions regarding the role of simple length of stay in determining treatment outcome (see above), is that the relationships shown between more counselling and lower likelihood of relapse to cocaine use were seen even among patients who completed treatment – that is, having approximately the same tenure in the programs. Thus, it may be that beyond the simple effects of attending a program, more involvement with the counselling activities is important for improved outcome.

At least four studies of substance abuse treatment have documented between-therapist differences in patient outcomes. These differences have emerged both among professional psychotherapists with doctoral level training and among paraprofessional counsellors. Luborsky et al. [177] found outcome differences in a variety of areas among nine professional therapists providing ancillary psychotherapy to methadone maintenance patients. McLellan et al. [178] found that assignment to one of five methadone maintenance counsellor resulted in significant differences in treatment progress over the following six months. Specifically, patients transferred to one counsellor achieved significant reductions in illicit drug use, unemployment, and arrests while concurrently reducing their average methadone dose. In contrast, patients transferred to another counsellor evidenced increased unemployment and illicit drug use while their average methadone dose went up. In a study of two different interventions for problem drinkers, Miller, Taylor, and West [179] found significant differences between paraprofessional therapists in the percentage of their patients who improved by six month follow-up. These percentages varied from 25% for the least effective therapist to 100% for the most effective therapist. Finally, McCaul et al. [180] reported significant differences in post treatment drinking rates and several other outcomes among alcohol dependent patients assigned to different individual counsellors within an alcohol treatment program.

There is much research that needs to be done in this area. Although it is relatively clear that therapists and counsellors differ considerably in the extent to which they are able to help their patients achieve positive outcomes, it is less clear what distinguishes more effective from less effective therapists. In an experimental study of two different therapist styles, Miller, Benefield, and Tonigan [181] found that a client centred approach emphasizing reflective listening was more effective for problem drinkers than a directive, confrontational approach. In a review of the literature on therapist differences in substance abuse treatment, Najavits and Weiss [182] concluded, "The only consistent finding has been that therapists' in-session interpersonal functioning is positively associated with greater effectiveness" (p. 683). Among indicators of interpersonal functioning were the ability to form a helping alliance [177], measures of the level of accurate empathy and a measure of "genuineness", "concreteness" and "respect" [183].

It should be noted that there are a variety of certification programs for counsellor (Committee on Addiction Rehabilitation (CARF) and Certified Addictions Counsellor (CAC)) as well as other professions treating substance dependent patients (American Society of Addiction Medicine; American Academy of Psychiatrists in Addiction; recent added certification for psychologists through the American Psychological Association). These "added qualification certificates" are offered throughout the country, usually by professional organizations. Although the efforts of these professional organizations to bring needed training and proficiency to the treatment of addicted persons are commendable, we were unable to find any studies validating whether patients treated by "certified" addictions counsellors, physicians or psychologists have better outcomes than patients treated by noncertified individuals. This is an important gap in the existing literature and results from such studies would be quite important for the licensing efforts and health policy decisions of many states and health care organizations.

Community reinforcement and contingency contracting

Azrin et al. initially developed the "Community Reinforcement Approach" (CRA) and tested it against other "standard" treatment interventions [184]. CRA includes conjoint therapy, job finding training, counselling focused on alcohol-free social and recreational activities, monitored disulfiram, and an alcohol-free social club. The goal of CRA is to make abstinence more rewarding than continued use [185]. In a study in which patients were randomly assigned to CRA or to a standard hospital treatment program, those getting CRA drank less, spent fewer days away from home, worked more days, and were institutionalized less over a 24 month follow-up [184].

A more recent set of studies by Higgins et al. [186-189] has used the CRA approach with cocaine dependent patients. Here, cocaine dependent patients seeking outpatient treatment were randomly assigned to receive either standard drug counselling and referral to AA, or a multi-component behavioural treatment integrating contingency managed counselling, community based incentives and family therapy comparable to the CRA model [189]. The CRA model retained more patients in treatment, produced more abstinent patients and longer periods of abstinence, and produced greater improvements in personal function than the standard counselling approach. Following the overall findings, this group of investigators systematically "disassembled" the CRA model and examined the individual "ingredients" of family therapy [188], incentives (Higgins et al., 1994), and the contingency based counselling [186] as compared against groups who received comparable amounts of all components except the target ingredient. In each case, these systematic and controlled examinations indicated that these individual components made a significant contribution to the outcomes observed, thus proving their added value in the rehabilitation effort.

"Matching" patients and treatments

There have been a great number of research studies attempting to "match" particular "kinds" of patients with specific types, modalities or settings of treatment. The approach to patient-treatment "matching" that has received the greatest attention from substance abuse treatment researchers involves attempting to identify the characteristics of individual patients that predict the best response to different forms of addiction treatments (e.g., cognitive-behavioral vs 12-Step, or inpatient *vs* outpatient) [169]. In general, the majority of these "patient-to-treatment" matching studies have *not* shown robust or generalizable findings [190]. Another approach to matching has been to assess patients' problem severity in a range of areas at intake and then "match" the specific and necessary services to the particular problems presented at the assessment. This has been called "problem-to-service" matching [191]. This approach may have more practical application as it is consonant with the "individually tailored treatment" philosophy that has been espoused by most practitioners.

Substance abusers with comorbid psychiatric problems may be particularly good candidates for the "problem-to-service" matching approach; especially the addition of specialized psychiatric services for those most severely affected by psychiatric problems. For example, recent studies suggest that tricyclic antidepressants and the selective serotonergic medication fluoxetine may reduce both drinking and depression levels in alcoholics with major depression [192-194]. Similarly, the anxiolytic buspirone may reduce drinking in alcoholics with a comorbid anxiety disorder [195]. Highly structured relapse prevention interventions may also be more effective in decreasing cocaine use, as compared to less structured interventions, in cocaine abusers with comorbid depression [196].

Woody *et al.* have evaluated the value of individual psychotherapy when added to paraprofessional counselling services in the course of methadone maintenance treatment [197]. In that study patients were randomly assigned to receive standard drug counselling alone (DC group) or drug counselling plus one of two forms of professional therapy: supportive-expressive psychotherapy (SE) or cognitive-behavioral psychotherapy (CB) over a six month period. Results showed that patients receiving psychotherapy showed greater reductions in drug use, more improvements in health and personal function and greater reductions in crime than those receiving counselling alone. Stratification of patients according to their levels of psychiatric symptoms at intake showed that the main psychotherapy effect was seen in those with greater than average levels of psychiatric symptoms. Specifically, patients with low symptom levels made considerable gains with counselling alone and there were no differences between types of treatment. However, patients with more severe psychiatric problems showed few gains with counselling alone but substantial improvements with the addition of the professional psychotherapy.

Another type of substance abuser that can pose particular problems for outpatient treatment is the cocaine dependent patient who is unable to achieve remission from cocaine dependence early in outpatient treatment. Several randomized studies suggest that highly structured cognitive-behavioral treatment is particularly efficacious with such individuals. In two outpatient studies with cocaine abusers, those with more severe cocaine problems at intake had significantly better cocaine use outcomes if they received structured relapse prevention rather than interpersonal or clinical management treatments [104, 149]. In a third study, cocaine dependent patients who continued to use cocaine during a four-week intensive outpatient treatment program (IOP) had much better cocaine use outcomes if they subsequently received aftercare that included a combination of group therapy and a structured relapse prevention protocol delivered through individual sessions rather than aftercare that consisted of group therapy alone [171].

McLellan *et al.* recently attempted to match "problems to services" in two inpatient and two outpatient private treatment programs [191]. Patients in the study (N = 130) were assessed with the ASI at intake and placed in a program that was acceptable to both the EAP referral source and the patient. At intake, patients were also randomized to either the standard or "matched" services conditions. In the standard condition, the treatment program received information from the intake ASI, and personnel were instructed to treat the patient in the "standard manner, as though there were no evaluation study ongoing". The programs were instructed to not withhold any services from patients in the standard condition. Patients who were randomly assigned to the matched services condition were also placed in one of the four treatment programs and ASI information was forwarded to that program. However, the programs agreed to provide at least three individual sessions in the areas of employment, family/social relations, or psychiatric health delivered by a professionally trained staff person. In fact, matched patients received significantly more psychiatric and employment services than standard patients, but not more family/social services or alcohol and drug services. Second, matched patients were more likely to complete treatment (93% *vs* 81%), and showed more improvement in the areas of employment and psychiatric functioning than the standard patients. Third, while matched and standard patients had sizable and equivalent improvements on most measures of alcohol and drug use, matched patients were less likely to be retreated for substance abuse problems during the six month follow-up. These findings suggest that matching treatment services to adjunctive problems can improve outcomes in key areas and may also be cost-effective by reducing the need for subsequent treatment due to relapse.

Summary of Part III

In Part III of this paper we briefly reviewed the substance abuse treatment research literature to identify treatment process variables and treatment components that have been shown to be important in determining outcome from addiction rehabilitation efforts; and in this way to contribute to the discussion of what aspects of treatment are "worth it" to society. The major treatment variables or components are summarized in *table* V below.

Table V. Components of effective treatment.

Treatment variables:
- Staying longer in treatment.
- Reinforcement (financial incentives or vouchers) for attendance and abstinence.
- Having an individual counselor or therapist.
- Specialized services for psychiatric, employment and family problems.
- Medications to:
  – Block drug craving and drug effects.
  – Reduce psychiatric symptoms.
- Participating in AA or NA following rehabilitation.

In light of these findings, it was surprising that some of the treatment elements that are most widely provided in substance abuse treatment have *not* been associated with better outcome. For example, our review of the literature has shown little indication that any of the following lead to better or longer lasting outcomes following treatment:

– alcohol/drug education sessions,
– general group therapy sessions – especially "confrontation" sessions,
– acupuncture sessions,
– patient relaxation techniques,
– treatment program accreditation or professional certification criteria.

Holder and Miller [159] have also reviewed the available research on the effectiveness of various treatment components in the alcohol rehabilitation field. These researchers also concluded that there are a number of therapeutic practises and procedures that remain prevalent in the field that have not *yet* shown indication of success.

In this regard *it is important to note* that "the absence of evidence" does not prove a treatment element is ineffective. Some of the treatment practises or conventions cited may actually have benefits for some patients or under some circumstances but we have found little support for these in the existing literature.

Part IV. Why aren't addiction treatments considered as effective as treatments for other illnesses? Implications for the delivery and evaluation of addiction treatment

In the previous parts of this paper we have examined the addiction treatment field from the perspective of its value to society. It would seem that our review would provide a relatively simple answer to what appears to be a direct question of cost and value. Yet it is not a direct question at all. We have tried to show that the reasonable expectations of a society regarding any form of intervention designed to "take care of the drug problem" must address many different issues, all typically related to the "addiction related" problems that are so frightening and costly to society. Multiple perspectives on outcome are not typical in evaluations of medical illnesses. In the treatment of most chronic illnesses "effective" treatments are expected to reduce symptoms, increase function and prevent relapse – especially costly relapse. Thus, as a final perspective on the issue of the effectiveness and worth of addiction treatments, we now consider an evaluation of the effectiveness of addiction treatments using the criteria typical for evaluations of other chronic illnesses.

Chronic illness/continuing care perspective: implications for treatment and evaluation

There are no "cures" for any of the chronic medical illnesses reviewed here. Yet it is interesting that despite rather comparable rates of compliance and relapse across all of the disorders examined, there is no serious argument as to whether the treatments for diabetes, hypertension or asthma are "effective" or whether they should be supported by contemporary health insurance. However, this issue is very much in question with regard to treatments for drug dependence [7, 12]. In this regard, it is interesting that the relatively high relapse rates among diabetic, hypertensive and asthmatic patients following cessation of their medications have been considered evidence of the *effectiveness* of those medications and of the need for compliance enhancement strategies. In contrast, relapses to drug and alcohol use following cessation of addiction treatments has often been considered evidence of treatment *failure*.

One major difference is that drug dependence treatments are not provided, evaluated or insured under the same assumptions that pertain to other chronic illnesses. Particularly important in this regard is that drug dependence treatments are rarely delivered under a continuing care model that would be appropriate for a chronic illness. Indeed, with the exception of methadone maintenance and AA/NA forms of treatment (parenthetically, among the most effective forms of treatment currently available) most contemporary treatments for drug dependence are acute care episodes. For example, it is common for a drug dependent individual to be admitted to a 30 to 90 day outpatient rehabilitation program, rarely accompanied by medical monitoring or medication. This period of treatment is typically followed by discharge with referral to "community sources". While the intentions and overall goals of addiction treatment might be conceptualized as ongoing by those in the treatment field, operationally addiction treatments are delivered in much the same way as one might treat a surgical patient following a joint replacement. Outcome evaluations are typically conducted six to twelve months *following treatment discharge*. A major (sometimes the exclusive) measure in all these evaluations is whether the patients had been continuously abstinent *since leaving treatment*.

Consider these goals and this treatment/evaluation strategy applied to a hypertension treatment regimen. Patients who meet diagnostic criteria for hypertension would be admitted to a 30-90 day outpatient "hypertension rehabilitation" program where they might receive medication, behavioural change therapy, dietary education, and an exercise regimen. Because of insurance limits and evaluation goals, the medication would be tapered during the last days of the treatment and the patients would be referred to community sources. The evaluation team would recontact the patient six months later and determine whether the patient had been *continuously normotensive throughout that post treatment period*. Only those patients that met this criterion would be considered "successfully treated". Obviously, this hypothetical treatment management strategy and its associated outcome evaluation approach are absurd for any chronic illness – including drug dependence.

■ Conclusions

Although science has made great progress over the past several years, we cannot yet fully account for the physiological and psychological processes that transform controlled, voluntary "use" of alcohol and/or other drugs into uncontrolled, involuntary "dependence" on these substances – and we cannot cure this condition once it has been contracted. But can we treat it "effectively" and would a societal investment in treatment provide an attractive return on the investment?

The research reviewed here suggests the answer is clearly yes to both parts of the question. Both controlled clinical trials and large-scale field studies have shown statistically and clinically significant improvements in drug use and in the drug-related health and social problems, of treated individuals. Further, these improvements translate into substantial reductions in social problems and costs to society. Recent pharmaceutical research has produced effective medications for the treatment of alcohol, nicotine and opiate dependence, and has identified promising candidate medications that will provide even more assistance to physicians in treating these illnesses. Thus, we conclude that drug and alcohol dependence are treatable medical illnesses.

If this conclusion is true, then why does it seem so surprising to so many parts of society. The thesis of this paper is that there are two main reasons for this.

Addiction is a chronic condition. Much of society has the view that addiction to drugs or alcohol is simply the product of poor impulse control complicated by the physiological problems associated with dependence and withdrawal. This assumption leads to a view that these acquired habits and withdrawal symptoms ought to be correctable with some education, some severe consequences associated with use (to teach the user a lesson) and some period of brief stabilization to "get the drugs out of their system". Our research is quite clear on these points, Education does not correct drug dependence – it is not simply a problem of lack of knowledge. Consequences for drug use appear to be important stimuli leading to drug abuse treatment entry. Indeed, over half of all treatment entrants in the United States are under some form of coercion [198]. At the same time, very few addicted individuals are able to profit from a corrections-oriented approach by itself. Relapse rates are over 70% to all forms of criminal justice interventions. Finally, addiction is not simply a matter of becoming stabilized and getting the drugs out of one's system. Relapse rates following detoxifications are approximately the same as those following incarceration [86, 94, 123, 153, 199].

The evidence is compelling that, at the present state of medical knowledge, addiction is best considered as a chronic relapsing condition. I have chosen the word "condition" for those who do not wish to call it an illness. It does not matter. Once considered a chronic condition it is no longer surprising that incarcerations, or brief stabilizations would not be effective. The research evidence is clear that for those with alcohol, cocaine, opiate or other drug dependence the best available treatments are those that are ongoing, able to address the multiple problems that are risks for relapse – such as medical and psychiatric symptoms and social instability – and are well integrated into society, thereby permitting ready access for monitoring purposes and to forestall relapse. Importantly, the research has shown that while motivation for treatment plays an important role in maintaining treatment participation – most substance abusing patients enter treatment with combinations of internal motivation and family, employment or legal pressure. These pressures can be combined with treatment interventions for the benefit of the patient and society.

Addiction Treatments Must Address the Concerns of Society. While we have compared addiction to other chronic illnesses, there are many differences. One of the most prominent differences is the breadth of treatment focus. The major foci of most treatments for other chronic illnesses are symptom remission and return of function for the benefit of the patient. This has also been true for many addiction treatments – and it has left much of society with the view that the major goal of addiction treatment is simply to make the patient feel better – not something those who have suffered from the crime, lost productivity and embarrassment of addiction are eager to do. Our perspective is that addiction treatment providers must broaden their views of their responsibilities. To achieve the potential social value of addiction treatment it will be necessary for providers to focus on such socially important goals as:

– working with employers and social welfare agencies toward the goals of returning to – or initiating work,
– working with criminal justice agencies and parole/probation officers toward the goals of keeping the patient from returning to drug-related crime and incarceration,
– working with family agencies and the families themselves toward the goals of returning to – or initiating responsible parenting.

These are the addiction-related conditions that most affect society. Reduction or elimination of these problems are the goals that society expects from any "effective" intervention. Our review has shown that addiction treatments can (but do not always) show evidence of being able to meet these societal expectations of effectiveness. With application of the treatment elements that have been shown to be effective under a continuing care model of treatment, our review suggests that addiction treatment can be an effective and valuable part of a social policy on drug abuse problems.

References

1. National Institute on Drug Abuse, *See how drug abuse takes the profit out of business*, Dept. of Health and Human Services USGPO, 1991.
2. Merrill J. *The cost of substance abuse to America's health care system, report 1: medicaid hospital hospital costs.* Center on Addiction and Substance Abuse, Columbia University, NY, 1993.
3. Rice DP, Kelman S, Miller LS. Estimates of the economic costs of alcohol, drug abuse and mental illness, 1985 and 1988. *Public Health Reports* 1991; 106 (3): 281-92.
4. Horgan C. *Chartbook of Social Indicators for Substance Abuse*. Princeton, NJ, Robert Wood Johnson Foundation Report, 1994.
5. Edelman MW. Children's Defense Fund Annual Report, Children's Defense Fund Press. 25 E. Street, Washington DC, 2001.
6. Saxe L, Dougherty D, Esty K, Fine M. *The Effectiveness and Costs of Alcoholism Treatment*. Health Technology Case Study 22. Office of Technology Assessment. Washington DC, 1983.
7. *Wall Street Journal*. Editorial Commentary, July 18, 1997: A12.
8. Fleming MF, Barry KL. The effectiveness of alcoholism screening in an ambulatory care setting. *J Stud Alcohol* 1991; 52: 33-6.
9. Schuckit MA. Why don't we diagnose alcoholism in our patients? *Journal of Family Practice* 1987; 25: 225-6.
10. Weisner CM, Schmidt L. Alcohol and drug problems among diverse health and social service populations. *American Journal of Public Health* 1993; 83: 824-9.
11. Conrad P, Schneider JW. *Deviance and Medicalization: From badness to sickness*. Toronto: CV Mosby Co, 1980.
12. *New York Times*, Editorial Section, November 20, 1997: A31.
13. Edwards G, Gross M. Alcohol dependence: provisional description of a clinical syndrome. *Br Med J* 1976; 1: 1058-61.
14. American Psychiatric Association. *Diagnostic and Statistical Manual of Mental Disorders*. Fourth Edition, 1994, Washington DC: APA Press.
15. Aceto MD, Scates SM, Lowe JA, Martin BR. Dependence on delta 9-tetrahydrocannabinol: Studies on precipitated and abrupt withdrawal. *J Pharmacol Exp Ther* 1996; 278: 1290-5.
16. Tsou DT, Patrick SL, Walder JM. Physical withdrawal in rats tolerant to delta 9-tetrahydrocannabinol precipitated by a cannabinoid receptor atagonist. *Eur J Pharmacol* 1995; 280: R13-5.
17. Hasin D, Grant BF, Cottler L, Blaine J, Towle L, et al. Nosological comparisons of alcohol and drug diagnoses: a multisite, multi-instrument international study. *Drug and Alcohol Dependence* 1997; 47: 217-26.
18. Rounsaville BJ, Kosten TR, Weissman MM, Prusoff B, Pauls D, Anton SF, et al. Psychiatric disorders in relatives of probands with opiate addiction. *Arch Gen Psychiat* 1991; 48 (1): 33-42.
19. Rounsaville BJ, Babor TF, Meyer RE. Psychiatric symptomatology in alcoholics. *Arch General Psychiat* 1989; 46: 45-51.
20. Smith TW, Turner CW, Ford MH, Hunt SC, Barlow GK, Stults BM, Williams RR. Blood pressure reactivity in adult male twins. *Health Psychology* 1987; 6 (3): 209-20.
21. Fagard R, Brguljan J, Staessen J, Thijs L, Derom C, Thomis M, Vlietinck R. Heritability of conventional and ambulatory blood pressures. A study in twins. *Hypertension* 1995; 26 (6 Pt 1): 919-24.

22. Hong Y, de Faire U, Heller DA, McClearn GE, Pedersen N. Genetic and environmental influences on blood pressure in elderly twins. *Hypertension* 1994; 24 (6): 663-70.
23. Kyvik KO, Green A, Beck-Nielsen H. Concordance rates of insulin dependent diabetes mellitus: a population based study of young Danish twins. *British Medical Journal* 1995; 311: 913-7.
24. Kaprio J, Tuomilehto J, Koskenvuo M, Romanov K, Reunanen A, Eriksson J, et al. Concordance for type 1 (insulin-dependent) and type 2 (non-insulin-dependent) diabetes mellitus in a population-based cohort of twins in Finland. *Diabetologia* 1992; 35 (11): 1060-7.
25. Duffy DL, Martin NG, Battistutta D, Hopper JL, Mathews JD. Genetics of asthma and hay fever in Australian twins. *Am Rev Respir Dis* 1990; 142 (6 Pt 1): 1351-8.
26. Nieminen MM, Kaprio J, Koskenvuo M. A population-based study of bronchial asthma in adult twin pairs. *Chest* 1991; 100 (1): 70-5.
27. Johnson EO, van den Bree M, Uhl GR, Pickens RW. Indicators of genetic and environmental influences in drug abusing individuals. *Drug and Alcohol Dependence* 1996; 41: 17-23.
28. Pickens RW, Elmer GI, LaBuda MC, Uhl GR. *Genetic Vulnerability to substance abuse.* Berlin: Springer Verlag, 1996.
29. Tsuang MT, Lyons MJ, Eisen S, Goldberg J, True W, Lin N, et al. Genetic influences on DSM-III-R drug abuse and dependence: A study of 3,372 twin pairs. *American Journal of Medical Genetics* 1996; 6 (7): 473-7.
30. Gynther LM, Carey G, Gottesman II, Vogler GP. A twin study of non-alcohol substance abuse. *Psychiatry Research* 1995; 56 (3): 213-20.
31. Kendler KS, Heath AC, Neale MC, Kessler RC, Eaves LJ. A population-based twin study of alcoholism in women. *Journal of the American Medical Association* 1992; 268: 1877-82.
32. Mitchell BD, Kammerer CM, Blangero J, Mahaney MC, Rainwater DL, Dyke B, et al. Genetic and environmental contributions to cardiovascular risk factors in Mexican Americans. The San Antonio Family Heart Study. *Circulation* 1996; 94 (9): 2159-70.
33. Svetkey LP, McKeown SP, Wilson AF. Heritability of salt sensitivity in black Americans. *Hypertension* 1996; 28 (5): 854-8.
34. Schuckit MA. Subjective responses to alcohol in sons of alcoholics and control subjects. *Arch Gen Psychiat* 1984; 41: 879-84.
35. Schuckit MA, Smith TL. An 8-year follow-up of 450 sons of alcoholics and controls. *Arch Gen Psychiat* 1996; 53: 202-10.
36. Thomasson HR, Edenberg HJ, Crabb DW, Mai XL, Jerome RE, Li TK, et al. Alcohol and aldehyde dehydrogenase genotypes and alcholism in Chinese men. *Am J Hum Genetics* 1991; 48: 667-81.
37. Helzer JE, Canino GJ, Yeh EK, Bland RC, Lee CK, Hwu HG, Newman S Alcoholism – North America and Asia. *Arch Gen Psychiat* 1990; 47: 313-9.
38. Chao YC, Kiou SR, Chung YY, Tang HS, Hsu CS, Li TK, Yin SJ. Polymorphism of alcohol and aldehyde dehydrogenase genes and alcoholic cirrhosis in Chinese patients. *Hepatology* 1994; 19: 360-6.
39. Koob GF, Bloom FE. Cellular and molecular mechanisms of drug dependence. *Science* 1988; 242: 715-23.
40. *Science* (1997) October 3 Issue. Volume 278, Issue 5335: 45-69.
41. *The Lancet* (1996) Special Issue on Addiction. Volume 347, Issue 9013: 1604-79.
42. National Academy of Sciences, Institute of Medicine. *Dispelling the Myths About Addiction.* Washington: National Academy Press, 1995.
43. Institute of Medicine. In: Fulco CE, Liverman CT, Earley LE, eds. *Development of Medications for the Treatment of Opiate and Cocaine Addictions: Issues for the Government and Private Sector.* Washington DC: National Academy Press, 1995.
44. Wise RA, Bozarth MA. Brain substrates for reinforcement and drug-self-administration. *Progress in Neuropsychopharmacology* 1981; 5: 467-74.
45. Volkow ND, Fowler JS, Wolf AP, Hitzemann R, Dewey S, Bendriem B, et al. Changes in brain glucose metabolism in cocaine dependence and withdrawal. *American Journal Psychiatry* 1991; 148 (5): 621-6.

46. London ED, Cascella NG, Wong DF, Phillips RL, Dannals RF, Links JM, et al. Cocaine-induced reduction of glucose utilization in human brain. A study of positron emission tomography and [flourine 18]-fluorodeoxyglucose. *Archives of General Psychiatry* 1990; 47: 567-74.

47. Weiss F. Neurochemical adaptation in brain reward systems during drug addiction. In: *Advancing Understanding of Drug Addiction*. Washington DC: National Academy of Sciences, 1996.

48. Kreek MJ, Koob GF. Drug dependence: stress and dysregulation of brain reward pathways. *Drug and Alcohol Dependence* 1998; 51 (1-2): 23-48.

49. Self DW, Nestler EJ. Drug dependence: stress and dysregulation of brain reward athways. *Drug and Alcohol Dependence* 1998; 51 (1-2): 49-60.

50. Roberts DCS, Corcoran ME, Fibiger HC. On the role of ascending catecholaminergic systems in intravenous self-administration of cocaine. *Pharmacology, Biochemistry and Behavior* 1977; 6: 615-20.

51. Phillips AG, Pfaus JG, Blaha CD. Dopamine and motivated behavior: insights provided by *in vivo* analyses. In: Willner P, Scheel-Kruger J, eds. *The Mesolimbic Dopamine System: From Motivation to Action*. John Wiley & Sons, 1995: 199-224.

52. Volkow ND. Relationship between subjective effects of cocaine and dopamine transporter occupancy. *Nature* 1997; 386 (6227): 827-30.

53. Volkow ND, Fowler JS, Wang G, Hitzemann R, Logan J, Schyler DJ, et al. Decreased dopamine D2 receptor availability is associated with reduced frontal metabolism in cocaine abusers. *Synapse* 1993; 14: 169-77.

54. Volkow ND, Hitzemann R, Wang GJ, Fowler JS, Wolf AP, Handelsman L. Long-term frontal brain metabolic changes in cocaine abusers. *Synapse* 1992; 11: 184-90.

55. Childress AR, McLellan AT, Ehrman R, O'Brien CP. Classically conditioned responses in opioid and cocaine dependence: a role in relapse? In: Ray B, ed. *Learning Factors in Substance Abuse, Research Monograph 84*. Washington DC: National Institute on Drug Abuse, 1988: 25-43.

56. Baxter LR, Schwartz JM, Phelps M. Localization of neurochemical effects of cocaine and other stimulants in the human brain. *J Clin Psychiatry* 1988; 49: 23-6.

57. Volkow ND, Mullani N, Gould KL, Adler S, Krajewski K. Cerebral blood flow in chronic cocaine users: a study with positron emission tomography. *British Journal of Psychiatry* 1988; 152: 641-8.

58. Holman BL, Mendelson J, Garada B, Teoh SK, Hallgring E, Johnson KA, et al. Regional cerebral blood flow improves with treatment in chronic cocaine polydrug users. *Journal Nuclear Medicine* 1993; 34: 723-7.

59. Pearlson GD, Jeffery PJ, Harris GJ, Ross CA, Fischman MW, Camargo EE. Correlation of acute cocaine-induced changes in local cerebral blood flow with subjective effects. *Am J Psychiatry* 1993; 150 (3): 495-7.

60. O'Brien CP. Experimental analysis of conditioning factors in human narcotic addiction. *Pharmacological Review* 1995; 27 (4): 533-43.

61. Childress AR, McElgin W, Mozley PD, Fitzgerald J, Reivich M, O'Brien CP. Limbic activation during cue-induced cocaine craving. *Am J Psychiatry* 1999; 156 (1): 11-8.

62. Stewart RG, Ware LG. *The Medical Outcomes Study*. The Rand Corp. Press, Santa Monica, California, 1989.

63. McLellan AT, Woody GE, Metzger D, McKay J, Alterman AI, O'Brien CP. Evaluating the Effectiveness of Treatments for Substance Use Disorders: Reasonable Expectations, Appropriate Comparisons. *The Milbank Quarterly* 1996; 74 (1): 51-85.

64. Ball JC, Ross A. *The Effectiveness of Methadone Maintenance Treatment*. New York: Springer-Verlag, 1991.

65. Food and Drug Administration, *Compliance Policy Guidelines*. Code of Federal Regulations. Volume 21, Paragraph 310. Washington DC, USGPO, 1990.

66. Metzger DS, Woody GE, McLellan AT, Druley P, DePhillipis D, O'Brien C, et al. HIV seroconversion among in and out of treatment intravenous drug users: An 18-month Prospective Follow-up. *AIDS* 1993; 6 (9): 1049-56.

67. Neaiguus A, Sufian M, Friedman SR. Effects of outreach intervention on risk reduction among intravenous drug users. *AIDS* 1990; 2: 253-71.

68. Booth R, Weibel WW. Effectiveness of reducing needle-related risk behaviors for HIV through indigenous outreach to injection drug users. *Am J Addictions* 1992; 23: 277-87.

69. Anderson MD, Smereck GA, Braunstein MS. LIGHT model: An effective intervention to change high-risk AIDS behavior among hard-to-reach urban drug users. *A J Drug and Alcohol Abuse* 1993; 19: 309-25.

70. McLellan AT, Metzger DS, Alterman AI, Woody GE, Durell J, O'Brien CP. Is addiction treatment "worth it"? Public health expectations, policy-based comparisons. In: Lewis DL, ed. *Proceedings of Josiah Macy Conference on Medical Education*. New York: Josiah Macy Foundation, 1995: 165-212.

71. Booth RE, Crowley TJ, Zhang Y. Substance abuse treatment entry, retention and effectiveness: out-of-treatment opiate injection drug users. *Drug and Alcohol Dependence* 1996; 42: 11-20.

72. Strecher VJ, Korbin SC, Kreuter MW, Roodhouse K, Farrel D. Opportunities for alcohol screening and counselling in primary care. *J Fam Practice* 1994; 39: 26-32.

73. Babor TF, Ritson EB, Hodgson RJ. Alcohol-related problems in the primary care setting: A review of early intervention strategies. *Br J Addiction* 1986; 81: 23-46.

74. Svikis DS, Golden AS, Huggins GR, Pickens RW, McCaul ME, et al. Cost effectiveness of treatment for drug abuseing pregnant women. *Drug and Alcohol Dependence* 1997; 45 (1, 2): 105-15.

75. Finnegan L, Kandall S. Maternal and neonatal effects of alcohol and drugs. In: Lowinson J et al., eds. *Substance Abyse: A Comprehensive Textbook* (Second Edition). Williams and Wilkins, 1992: 628-56.

76. Glantz JK, Woods JR. Cocaine, heroin and phyencyclidine: Obstetric perspectives. *Clin Obstet Gynecol* 1993; 85: 468-79.

77. Haller DL, Knisely JS, Dawson KS, Schnoll SH. Perinatal substance abusers: Psychological and psychosocial characteristics. *J Nerv Ment Dis* 1993; 18: 509-13.

78. Philbbs CS, Batema DA, Schwartz RM. The neonatal costs of maternal cocaine use. *JAMA* 1991; 11: 1521-6.

79. Anton RF. New Directions in the pharmacotherapy of alcoholism. *Psychiatric Annals* 1995; 25: 353-62.

80. O'Brien CP. Recent developments in the pharmacotherapy of substance abuse. *Journal of Consulting and Clinical Psychology* 1996; 64: 677-86.

81. Nightingale SL. Levomethadyl approved for the treatment of opiate dependence. *JAMA* 1993; 270: 1290.

82. Milby JB. Methadone maintenance to abstinence. How many make it? *J Nerv Ment Dis* 1988; 176: 409-22.

83. McCance-Katz EF, Kosten TR. *New treatments for chemical addictions*. Washington: APP, 1998.

84. Gossop M, Johns A, Green L. Opiate withdrawal: inpatient *versus* outpatient programmes and preferred *versus* random assignment. *British Medical Journal* 293: 103-4.

85. Mattick RP, Hall W. Are detoxification programmes effective? *Lancet* 1996; 347: 97-100.

86. National Consensus Development Panel. Effective Medical Treatment of Opiate Addiction: Report of the NIH Consensus Conference on the Treatment of Opiate Addiction. *JAMA* 1998; 280 (22): 1936-43.

87. Bickel WK, Amass L. Buprenorphine treatment of opioid dependence: A review. *Experimental and Clinical Psychopharmacology* 1995; 3: 477-89.

88. Johnson RE, Cone EJ, Henningfield JE, Fudala PJ. Use of buprenorphine in the treatment of opioid addiction. *Clinical Pharmacology and Therapeutics* 1989; 46: 335-43.

89. O'Brien CP, Childress AR, McLellan AT, Ternes J, Ehrman R. Use of naltrexone to extinguish opioid conditioned responses. *Journal of Clinical Psychiatry* 1984; 45 (9): 53-6.

90. Resnick RB, Volavka J, Freedman AM, Thomas M. Studies of EN-1639-A (naltrexone): A new narcotic antagonist. *Am J Psychiatry* 1974; 131: 646-50.

91. O'Brien CP, Greenstein RA, Mintz J, Woody GE. Clinical experience with naltrexone. *American Journal of Drug & Alcohol Abuse* 1975; 2: 365-77.

92. Martin WR, Jasinski DR, Mansky PA. Naltrexone, an antagonist for the treatment of heroin dependence. *Archives of General Psychiatry* 1973; 28: 784-91.

93. Ling W, Wesson DR. Naltrexone treatment for addicted health care professionals: A collaborative private practise experience. *J Clin Psychiat* 1984; 45 (9): 46-8.

94. Cornish J, Metzger D, Woody G, et al. Naltrexone pharmacotherapy for opioid dependent federal probationers. *J SubstanceAbuse Treatment* 1998; 13: 477-89.

95. Volpicelli JR, Alterman AI, Hayashida M, O'Brien CP. Naltrexone in the treatment of alcohol dependence. *Arch Gen Psychiat* 1992; 49: 876-80.

96. O'Malley SS, Jaffe AJ, Chang G, et al. Naltrexone and coping skills therapy for alcohol dependence: A controlled study. *Arch Gen Psychiat* 1992; 49: 881-7.

97. Sass H, Soyka M, Mann K, Zieglgasberger W. Relapse prevention by acamprosate: results from a placebo-controlled study on alcohol dependence. *Arch Gen Psychiat* 1996; 53: 673-80.

98. Fox BS. Development of a therapeutic vaccine for the treatment of cocaine addiction. *Drug and Alcohol Dependence* 1997; 48: 153-8.

99. Woody GE, O'Brien CP, Rickels K. Depression and anxiety in heroin addicts: A placebo-controlled study of doxepin in combination with methadone. *Am J Psychiatry* 1975; 132 (4): 447-50.

100. Carroll KM, Rounsaville BJ, Gordon LT, Nich C, Jatlow P, Bisighini RM, Gawin FH. Psychotherapy and pharmacotherapy for ambulatory cocaine abusers. *Archives of General Psychiatry* 1994; 51: 177-87.

101. Mason BJ, Kocsis JH, Ritvo EC, Cutler RB. A double-blind, placebo-controlled trial of desipramine for primary alcohol dependence stratified on the presence or absence of major depression. *Journal of the American Medical Association* 1996; 275: 761-7.

102. Kosten TR, Rounsaville BJ, Kleber HD. Multidimensionality and prediction and treatment outcome in opioid addicts: 2.5-year follow-up. *Comprehensive Psychiatry* 1987; 28: 3-13.

103. Rounsaville BJ, Dolinsky ZS, Babor TF, Meyer RE. Psychopathology as a predictor of treatment outcome in alcoholics. *Archives of General Psychiatry* 1987; 44: 505-13.

104. Carroll KM, Power MD, Bryant K, Rounsaville BJ. One-year follow-up status of treatment-seeking cocaine abusers: Psychopathology and dependence severity as predictors of outcome. *Journal of Nervous and Mental Disease* 1993; 181: 71-9.

105. Babor TF. Brief intervention strategies for harmful drinkers: New directions for medical education. *Canadian Medical Association Journal* 1990; 143: 1070-6.

106. Healther N, Campion PD, Neville RG, McCabe D. Evaluation of a controlled drinking minimal intervention for problem drinkers in general practise. *General Practice* 1987; 37: 358-63.

107. Miller WR. Techniques to modify hazardous drinking patterns. *Recent Developments in Alcohol* 1987; 5: 425-38.

108. Kristenson H, Ohlin H, Hulten-Nosslin M, Trell E, Hood B. Identification and intervention of heavy drinking in middle-aged men. *Alcoholism: Clinical and Experimental Research* 1983; 7: 203-9.

109. Wallace P, Cutler S, Haines A. Randomized controlled trial of general practitioner intervention in patients with excessive alcohol consumption. *British Medical Journal* 1988; 297: 663-8.

110. World Health Organization Brief Intervention Study Group. A Cross-national trial of brief intervention with heavy drinkers. *Am J Pub Health* 1996; 86: 948-55.

111. Fleming MF, Barry KL, Manwell LB, Johnson K, London R. Brief physician advice for problem alcohol drinkers: A randomized controlled trial in community-based primary care practise. *JAMA* 1997; 277: 1039-45.

112. Bien TH, Miller WR, Tonigan JS. Brief interventions for alcohol problems: A review. *Addiction* 1993; 88: 315-35.

113. Fleming MF, Mundt MP, French MT, Manwell LB, Stafffacher EA, Barry LB. Benefit-Cost analyses of brief physician advice with problem drinkers in primary care settings. *Medical Care* 2000; 38: 7-18.

114. Moos RH, Finney JW, Cronkite RC. *Alcoholism Treatment: Context, Process and Outcome.* New York: Oxford Univ. Press, 1990.

115. Simpson D, Savage L. Drug abuse treatment readmissions and outcomes. *Arch Gen Psychiat* 1980; 37: 896-901.

116. Hubbard RL, Marsden ME, Rachal JV, Harwood HJ, Cavanaugh ER, Ginzburg HM. *Drug Abuse Treatment: A National Study of Effectiveness.* Chapel Hill: Univ. of North Carolina Press, 1989.

117. DeLeon G. The Therapeutic Community: Study of Effectiveness *Treatment Research Monograph 84-1286.* Rockville, Md: NIDA, 1984.

118. Miller WR, Hester RK. The Effectiveness of Alcoholism Treatment Methods: What Research Reveals. In: Miller WR, Heather N, eds. *Treating Addictive Behaviors: Process of Change*. New York: Plenum Press, 1986.
119. Gerstein D, Harwood H, eds. *Treating Drug Problems* (Volume One). Washington DC: National Academy Press, 1990.
120. Gerstein D, Judd LL, Rovner SA. Career dynamics of female heroin addicts. *Am J Drug and Alc Abuse* 1979; 6 (1): 1-23.
121. McLellan AT, Alterman AI, Metzger DS, Grissom G, Woody GE, Luborsky L, O'Brien CP. Similarity of Outcome Predictors Across Opiate, Cocaine and Alcohol Treatments: Role of Treatment Services. *J Clin Consult Psychol* 1984; 62 (6): 1141-58.
122. Volpicelli JR, Rhines KC, Rhines JS, Volpicelli LA, Alterman AI, O'Brien CP. Naltrexone and alcohol dependence. Role of subject compliance. *Archives of General Psychiatry* 1997; 54 (8): 737-42.
123. McLellan AT, Woody GE, Metzger D, McKay J, Alterman AI, O'Brien CP. Evaluating the Effectiveness of Treatments for Substance Use Disorders: Reasonable Expectations, Appropriate Comparisons. *The Milbank Quarterly* 1996; 74 (1): 51-85.
124. O'Brien CP, McLellan AT. Myths about the treatment of addiction. *Lancet* 1996; 347: 237-40.
125. Graber AL, Davidson P, Brown A, McRae J, Woolridge K. Dropout and relapse during diabetes care. *Diabetic Care* 1992; 15 (11): 1477-83.
126. Horowitz RI. Treatment adherence and risk of death after a myocardial heart infarction. *Lancet* 1993; 336 (8714): 542-5.
127. Dekker FW, Dieleman FE, Kaptein AA, Mulder JD. Compliance with pulmonary medication in general practise. *European Respiratory Journal* 1993; 6 (6): 886-90.
128. Clark LT. Improving compliance and incrasing control of hypertension: Needs of special hypertensive populations. *American Heart Journal* 1991; 121 (2 Pt 2): 664-9.
129. Kurtz SM. Adherence to diabetic regimes: Empirical status and clinical applications. *Diabetes Education* 1990; 16 (1): 50-9.
130. Sinnock P. Hospitalization of diabetes. In *Dabetes Data*, National Diabetes Data Group, Bethesda Md., National Institutes of Health, 1985.
131. Herman WH, Teutsch SM. Diabetic renal disorders. In *Diabetes Data*, National Diabetes Data Group, Bethesda Md., National Institutes of Health, 1985.
132. Schaub AF, Steiner A, Vetter W. Compliance to treatment. *Journal of Clinical and Experimental Hypertension* 1993; 15 (6): 1121-30.
133. Gorlin R. Hypertension and ischemic heart disease: The challenge of the 1990s. *American Heart Journal* 1991; 121 (2 Pt 2): 658-63.
134. Satel SL, Price LH, Palumbo JM, McDougle CJ, et al. Clinical phenomenology and neurobiology of cocaine abstinence: A prospective inpatient study. *Am J Psychiatry* 1991; 148: 1712-6.
135. Weddington WW. Cocaine abstinence: ??Òwithdrawal??Ó or residua of chronic intoxication? *Am J Psychiatry* 1992; 149: 1761-2.
136. Gawin FH, Kleber HD. Abstinence symptomatology and psychiatric diagnoses in cocaine abusers. *Arch Gen Psychiat* 1986; 43: 107-13.
137. Gawin FH, Ellinwood EH. Cocaine and other stimulants: Actions, abuse, and treatment. *New Engl J Med* 1998; 318: 1173-82.
138. Fleming MF, Barry KL. *Addictive Disorders*. St. Louis: Mosby Yearbook Primary Care Series, 1992.
139. Hayshida M, Alterman AI, McLellan AT, et al. Comparitive effectiveness of inpatient and outpatient detoxification patient with mild-to-moderate alcohol withdrawal syndrome. *New Engl J Med* 1989; 320: 358-65.
140. Stockwell T, Bolt L, Milner I, Puch P, Young I. Home detoxification for problem drinkers: acceptability to clients, relatives, general practioners and outcome after 60 days. *British Journal of Addiction* 1990; 85: 61-70.
141. Legarda J. Ultra-rapid opiate detoxification. *Lancet* 2000; 351 (9014): 1517.

142. Brewer C, Williams J, Carreno-Rendueles E, Bobes-Garcia J. Unethical promotion of rapid opiate detoxification under anaesthesia (RODA). *Lancet* 2001; 351 (9097): 218.
143. Cushman P, Dole VP. Detoxification of rehabilitatied methadone-maintained patients. *JAMA* 1973; 226: 747-52.
144. Institute of Medicine. Federal Regulation of Methadone Treatment. Washington DC: National Academy Press, 1995.
145. Gossop M, Johns A, Green L. Opiate withdrawal: inpatient *versus* outpatient programmes and preferred *versus* random assignment. *British Medical Journal* 1986; 293: 103-4.
146. Lipton DS, Maranda MJ. Detoxification from heroin dependency: an overview of method and effectiveness. *Advances in Alcohol and Substance Abuse* 1983; 2: 31-55.
147. Alterman A, McKay J, Mulvaney F, McLellan AT. Prediction of attrition from day hospital treatment in lower socioeconomic cocaine-dependent men. *Drug and Alc Dep* 1996; 40: 227-33.
148. Kang SY, Kleinman PH, Woody GE, Millman RB, et al. Outcomes for cocaine abusers after once-a-week psychosocial therapy. *Am J Psychiatry* 1991; 148: 630-5.
149. Carroll KM, Rounsaville BJ, Gawin FH. A comparative trial of psychotherapies for ambulatory cocaine abusers: Relapse prevention and interpersonal psychotherapy. *American Journal of Drug & Alcohol Abuse* 1991; 17: 229-47.
150. Volpicelli JR, Alterman AI, Hayashida M, O'Brien CP. Naltrexone in the treatment of alcohol dependence. *Archives of General Psychiatry* 1992; 49: 876-80.
151. O'Malley SS, Jaffe AJ, Rode S, Rounsaville BJ. Experience of a "slip" among alcoholics treated with naltrexone or placebo. *Am J Psychiatry* 1996; 153: 281-3.
152. McLellan AT, Ball JC. Is Methadone Treatment Effective? In: Rettig R, ed. *A Re-Evaluation of Federal Regulations on Methadone Treatment*. Washington DC: Institute of Medicine Press, 1995.
153. McLellan AT, Woody GE, Metzger D, McKay J, Alterman AI, O'Brien CP. Evaluating the Effectiveness of Treatments for Substance Use Disorders: Reasonable Expectations, Appropriate Comparisons. In: Fox D, ed. *The Milbank Foundation Volume on Health Policy Issue*. New York: Milbank Foundation Press, 1995.
154. McLellan AT, Weisner C. Achieving the public health potential of substance abuse treatment: Implications for Patient Referral, Treatment "Matching" and Outcome Evaluation. In: Bickel W, DeGrandpre R, eds. *Drug Policy and Human Nature*. Philadelphia: Wilkins and Wilkins, 1996.
155. McLellan AT, Durell J. Evaluating Substance Abuse and Psychiatric Treatments: Conceptual and Methodological Considerations. In: Sederer L, ed. *Outcomes Assessment in Clinical Practice*. New York: Williams and Wilkins, 1995.
156. Alterman AI, McLellan AT, O'Brien CP, August DS, Snider EC, Cornish JC, et al. Effectiveness and Costs of Inpatient *Versus* Day Hospital Cocaine Rehabilitation. *J Nerv Ment Dis* 1994; 182: 157-63.
157. McCrady BS, Noel NE, Abrams DB, Stout RL, Nelson HF, Hay WM. Comparative effectiveness of three types of spouse involvement in outpatient behavioural alcoholism treatment. *J Studies on Alcohol* 1986; 47: 459-67.
158. Miller WR, Hester RK. Inpatient alcoholism treatment: Who benefits? *American Psychologist* 1986; 41: 794-805.
159. Holder HD, Longabaugh R, Miller WR, Rubonis A. The cost effectiveness of treatment for alcohol problems: A first approximation. *Journal of Studies on Alcohol* 1991; 52: 517-40.
160. Walsh DC, Hingson R, Merrigan D, et al. A randomized trial of treatment options for alcohol-abusing workers. *N Eng J Med* 1991; 325: 775-82.
161. Finney JW, Hahn AC, Moos RH. The effectiveness of inpatient and outpatient treatment of substance abuse: The need to focus on mediators and moderators of setting effects. *Addiction* 1996; 91: 1773-96.
162. McKay JR, Alterman AI, McLellan AT, Snider C, et al. Treatment goals, continuity of care, and outcome in a day hospital substance abuse rehabilitation program. *American Journal of Psychiatry* 1994; 151: 254-9.
163. McKay JR, McLellan AT, Alterman AI. An evaluation of the Cleveland Criteria for Inpatient Treatment of Substance Abuse. *Am J Psychiat* 1992; 149: 1212-8.

164. Ball JC, Ross A. *The Effectiveness of Methadone Maintenance Treatment.* New York: Springer-Verlag, 1991.
165. DeLeon G. *The Therapeutic Community: Study of Effectiveness Treatment Research Monograph #84-1286.* NIDA, Rockville, Md, 1984.
166. Hubbard RL, Marsden ME, Rachal JV, Harwood HJ, Cavanaugh ER, Ginzburg HM. Drug Abuse Treatment: A National Study of Effectiveness. Chapel Hill: Univ. of North Carolina Press, 1989.
167. Simpson DD. Treatment for drug abuse: Follow-up outcomes and length of time spent. *Archives of General Psychiatry* 1981; 38: 875-80.
168. Simpson DD, Joe GW, Brown BS. Treatment retention and follow-up outcomes in the Drug Abuse Treatment Outcome Study (DATOS). *Psychology of Addictive Behaviors* 1997; 11 (4): 294-301.
169. Project MATCH Research Group. Matching alcoholism treatments to client heterogeneity: Project MATCH posttreatment drinking outcomes. *Journal of Studies on Alcohol* 1997; 58: 7-29.
170. McLatchie BH, Lomp KG. Alcoholics Anonymous affiliation and treatment outcome among a clinical sample of problem drinkers. *American Journal of Drug & Alcohol Abuse* 1988; 14: 309-24.
171. McKay JR, Alterman AI, Cacciola JS, Rutherford MR, O'Brien CP, Koppenhaver J. Group counselling vs individualized relapse prevention aftercare following intensive outpatient treatment for cocaine dependence: Initial results. *Journal of Consulting and Clinical Psychology* 1997; 65: 778-88.
172. Timko C, Moos RH, Finney JW, Moos BS. Outcome of treatment for alcohol abuse and involvement in Alcoholics Anonymous among previously untreated problem drinkers. *Journal of Mental Health Administration* 1994; 21: 145-60.
173. Tonigan JS, Toscova R, Miller WR. Meta-analysis of the literature on Alcoholics Anonymous: Sample and study characteristics moderate findings. *Journal of Studies on Alcohol* 1996; 57: 65-72.
174. Morgenstern J, Labouvie E, McCrady B, Kahler C, Fre R. Affiliation with Alcoholics Anonymous following treatment: A study of its therapeutic effects and mechanisms of action. *Journal of Consulting and Clinical Psychology* 2001; 167: 85-92.
175. McLellan AT, Arndt IO, Woody GE, Metzger D. Psychosocial Services in Substance Abuse Treatment?: A dose-ranging study of psychosocial services. *J Am Med Assn* 1993; 269 (15): 1953-9.
176. Fiorentine R, Anglin MD. Does increasing the opportunity for counselling increase the effectiveness of outpatient drug treatment? *American Journal of Drug and Alcohol Abuse* 1997; 23 (3): 369-82.
177. Luborsky L, McLellan AT, Woody GE, O'Brien CP. Therapist success and its determinants. *Arch Gen Psych* 1985; 42: 602-11.
178. McLellan AT, Woody GE, Luborsky L, Goehl L. Is the counsellor an "active ingredient" in substance abuse rehabilitation? *Journal of Nervous and Mental Disease* 1988; 176: 423-30.
179. Miller WR, Taylor CA, West JC. Focused *versus* broad-spectrum behavior therapy for problem drinkers. *Journal of Consulting and Clinical Psychology* 1980; 48: 590-601.
180. McCaul M, Svikis D. Improving client compliance in outpatient treatment: Counselor-targeted interventions. *National Institute on Drug Abuse Research Monograph* 1991; 106: 204-17.
181. Miller WR, Benefiield RG, Tonigan JS. Enhancing motivation for change in problem drinking: A controlled comparison of two therapist styles. *Journal of Consulting and Clinical Psychology* 1993; 61: 455-61.
182. Najavits LM, Weiss RD. Variations in therapist effectiveness in the treatment of patients with substance use disorders: An empirical review. *Addiction* 1994; 89 (6): 679-88.
183. Valle S. Interpersonal functioning of alcoholism counsellor and treatment outcome. *Journal of Studies on Alcohol* 1981; 42: 783-90.
184. Azrin NH, Sisson RW, Meyers RW, Godley M. Alcoholism treatment by disulfiram and community reinforcement therapy. *Journal of Behavior Therapy and Experimental Psychiatry* 1982; 13: 105-12.
185. Meyers RJ, Smith JE. *Clinical guide to alcohol treatment: The Community Reinforcement Approach.* New York: Guilford, 1995.
186. Higgins ST, Budney AJ, Bickel WK, Badger GJ, Foerg FE, Ogden D. Outpatient behavioural treatment for cocaine dependence: One-year outcome. *Experimental and Clinical Psychopharmacology* 1995; 3: 205-12.

187. Higgins ST, Budney AJ, Bickel WK, Foerg FE, Donham R, Badger GJ. Incentives improve outcome in outpatient behavioural treatment of cocaine dependence. *Archives of General Psychiatry* 1994; 51: 568-76.
188. Higgins ST, Budney AJ, Bickel WK, Hughes JR, Foeg FE, Badger GJ. Achieving cocaine abstinence with a behavioural approach. *American Journal of Psychiatry* 1993; 150: 763-9.
189. Higgins ST, Delaney DD, Budney AJ, Bickel WK, Hughes JR, Foerg F, Fenwick JW. A behavioural approach to achieving initial cocaine abstinence. *Am J Psychiat* 1991; 148: 1218-24.
190. Gastfriend D, McLellan AT. Treatment Matching: Theoretical Basis and Practical Implications. In: Samet J, Stein M, eds. *Medical Clinics of North America*. New York: WB Saunders, 1997.
191. McLellan AT, Grissom G, Zanis D, Brill P. Problem – Service "Matching" In Addiction Treatment: A prospective study in four programs. *Arch Gen Psychiatry* 1997; 54: 730-5.
192. Cornelius JR, Salloum IM, Ehler JG, Jarrett PJ, Cornelius MD, Perel JM, et al. Fluoxetine in depressed alcoholics: A double-blind, placebo controlled trial. *Archives of General Psychiatry* 1997; 54: 700-5.
193. Mason BJ, Kocsis JH, Ritvo EC, Cutler RB. A double-blind, placebo-controlled trial of desipramine for primary alcohol dependence stratified on the presence or absence of major depression. *Journal of the American Medical Association* 1996; 275: 761-7.
194. McGrath PJ, Nunes EV, Stewart JW, Goldman D, Agosti V, Ocepek-Welikson K, Quitkin FM. Imipramine treatment of alcoholics with primary depression: A placebo-controlled clinical trial. *Archives of General Psychiatry* 1996; 53: 232-40.
195. Kranzler HR, Burleson JA, Del Boca FK, Babor TF, Korner P, Brown J, et al. Buspirone treatment of anxious alcoholics: A placebo-controlled trial. *Archives of General Psychiatry* 1994; 51: 720-31.
196. Carroll KM, Nich C, Rounsaville BJ. Differential symptom reduction in depressed cocaine abusers treated with psychotherapy and pharmacotherapy. *Journal of Nervous and Mental Disease* 1995; 183: 251-9.
197. Woody GE, McLellan AT, Luborsky L, et al. Psychiatric severity as a predictor of benefits from psychotherapy. *Am J Psychiat* 1984; 10: 1171-7.
198. Belenko S. *Behind Bars: Substance abuse and America's prison population*. New York: National Center for Addiction and Substance Abuse at Columbia University, 1998. www.casacolumbia.org.
199. Inciardi JA. Some considerations on the clinical efficacy of compulsory treatment: Reviewing the New York experience. In: Leukefeld CG, Tims FM, eds. *Compulsory Treatment of Drug Abuse: Research and Clinical Practice*. NIDA Research Monograph 86, 1988.

The British experience of dual diagnosis in the national health service

A. Lowe[1], M. T. Abou-Saleh[2]

1. Consultant Psychiatrist, St George's Hospital Medical School
2. Reader in Addiction Psychiatry, University of London, UK

The issue of "Dual Diagnosis" or comorbidity of serious mental illness and substance misuse problems has emerged as a major public health concern in the UK [1]. It occupies a place on the boundary between mainstream psychiatry and addiction services. The majority of the research work on service models derives from the USA, Canada or Australia and from these systems that in places have been running for several years we are urged to adopt a model of integrated service provision. Drake *et al.* [2] have demonstrated the effectiveness of the integrated model of service guided by evidence-based interventions. The integrated model has emerged from the failure of the traditional sequential or parallel models in which the patient fell through the'cracks'and lost in the borderland. As a result integrated services have been established in the form of Dual Diagnosis programmes. However the development of such programmes in the UK is not consistent with the NHS structure and the organisation of health and social services [3].

■ Two Different Views

Another difficult area to consider is the difference in philosophies between traditional addiction services and mental health. In addiction services the patient (more usually called client) is responsible for their own behaviour and can leave an interview or walk out of a residential rehabilitation setting if they so wish. In a mental health context if a practitioner is concerned (for example about the nature and severity of psychotic symptoms) common law or the mental health act may be used to stop a patient leaving. Indeed patients with a wide range of conditions from anorexia to schizophrenia may be admitted against their wishes for assessment and treatment under the Mental Health Act if they are found to be at sufficient risk. Admission for treatment for addiction alone is specifically excluded from the current act [4]. As a general principle, the mental health practitioner is more likely to assume a responsibility for a patient and intervene than an addictions worker is. The addiction field has embraced the motivational Interviewing as described by Miller and Rollnick [5]. The component of our role is about persuading and empowering patients to make changes against the apparent odds. The distance between philosophical stance may be decreasing as treatment options in the UK and now are increasingly being linked to the criminal justice system. The introduction of Drug Treatment and Testing Orders remains a controversial area but has introduced the idea of compulsion into treatment for Drug (but not alcohol) problems. Mental health is using motivational interviewing to help with compliance and the skills in the fields are becoming more complimentary and closely aligned.

The Evidence base/Health care system

The UK healthcare system is anchored in General Practice and promises to supply free care at point of delivery. In the UK, patients are not used to the idea of belonging to a programme or to the idea that entry to a programme would then provide funding for this "episode" of care. The Dual Diagnosis Program described by Drake et al. [2], that is able to take patients in, provide all their health care needs and hold onto them for up to five years, is not a viable option in resource terms or in context of current healthcare planning.

The National Service Framework (NSF) for Mental Health, whilst emphasising the importance of tackling dual diagnosis, has failed to provide standards and service models to address the challenges posed by this group of patients, including those with serious mental illness. It is against this background of policy gap that the Dual Diagnosis Good Practice Guide has been recently launched. Moreover the NSF has not provided standards and service models for people with substance misuse, requiring the development of complementary guidance on Models of Care which has been recently launched by the National Treatment Agency as the National Service Framework for Addictions. The key message in this Guide is that substance misuse is usual rather than exceptional among people with serious mental health problems and that the relationship between the two disorders is complex. Individuals with dual diagnosis have varied and complex needs and require high quality, comprehensive and integrated care that should be delivered within mainstream mental health services. The Guide recognises that *mainstreaming* will not reduce the role of drug and alcohol services which will continue to treat the majority of people with substance misuse problems and advise on substance misuse issues. The Guide summarises good practise in relation to treatment and sets out a programme for local implementation of the appropriate service model. It is concluded that in integrated care – carried out by one team – delivers better outcomes than serial care (sequential referrers to different services) or parallel care (more than one service engaging a patient at the same time). The approach chosen was to bridge the gaps not by another free standing service but by trying to develop a responsive, flexible service to help patients access care in networks that already exist. The service works as an adjunct to the care the patient already has and is not a substitute for other services remaining or becoming involved.

The guidance is timely and welcome and in so far as it focuses on the needs of patients with serious mental illness and co-morbid substance misuse it is a step in the right direction. It places lead responsibility with mainstream mental health services: provides joined-up thinking at the policy level, standards of good practise in assessment and treatment with good examples such as the Kingston Community Drug and Alcohol Team, the Haringey Dual Diagnosis Service and the COMPASS Programme in Birmingham; guidance on implementation and commissioning standards. However the guidance fails to address important issues relating to social care, the resource implications of this major service development, the interface between mainstream mental health services and addiction services as well as the implications for the future of and the scope of addiction services.

Concerning social care, particularly the housing needs of this vulnerable population, there is a distinct lack of provision of social care with the very limited access to mainstream community care and residential care facilities in mental health and addiction. This is a prime task for Local Implementation Teams working with Drug Action Teams to tackle this problem. This is also important as the pooled budget for drug misuse is targeted to the increased treatment for the rising demand for drug misuse services and whether mainstream mental health funding could cater for the needs of this population. A most important implication of this guidance is the role of addiction services vis-à-vis mainstream mental health services which lack capacity to deal with this population. A survey of the training and support needs of staff working with patients dual diagnosis showed that staff within mental health services lacked knowledge and skills for assessment and treatment of substance misuse and of the available resources and how to access substance misuse services. The role of addiction services is paramount in providing training and support for development of capacity and importantly in sustaining this capacity with optimal supervision and the agreement of local shared care working arrangements and care pathways, including the care programme approach. Our local experience at South West London and St George's Mental Health NHS Trust has been a positive one with the introduction of shared care working arrangements and protocol, which provided also for optimum access to mental health services for assessment and treatment of patients with dual diagnosis, who access addiction services. However, one problem that has persisted is that of those with substance-induced psychiatric disorders, those with high risk of self harm and harm to others who are often not accepted by mainstream mental health services. From the perspective of addiction services, the introduction and the implementation of the Models of Care framework could address these difficulties: commissioners and providers of services should consider how to integrate these two sets of guidance, which will also provide clarity for the interface of those referred to services from primary care.

Challenges to integration

Funding and diversity

The funding arrangements are very different in the UK as compared to the US. The state funding of the National Health Service and the way specialised services are commissioned have not enabled a system where funding truly follows the patients and meets their needs. Dual Diagnosis patients particularly those at the severe end of the spectrum with serious mental illness are in contact with highly stretched national health funded psychiatric services. They have multiple needs of mental health; addiction and social care but may find access difficult or become excluded due to aspects of behaviour. The budget streams of these services are in different places although we are moving towards integrated "Health Care Trusts". Whilst we may integrate health and social Services at a secondary and tertiary level these patients still have needs such as housing which have to be integrated into their care plans. Primary care in the UK is the gatekeeper unlike the situation in the USA and the purchasing power of Primary Care Trusts may also influence how these patients are provided for. Addiction Services are purchased in England through Drug Action Teams (DAT), which may not consider Dual Diagnosis as priority as they are primed to respond to the drivers that come from the National Treatment Agency and central government around crime and disorder and drugs. Thus even at the planning stage in the UK trying to integrate care for these patients with the diversity of organisations involved remains complicated and challenging.

Responsibility and risk

Addiction and mental health operate under different philosophies in the UK. In addiction services the patient is free to leave treatment if they choose. Under the psychological models of harm minimisation and the cycle of change it is expected that there will be relapse and a process of reengagement afterwards. In a mental health interview there is always the question of whether a patient needs assessment for detention under the mental health act for their safety or that of others.

The mental health act does not have a provision for detaining a patient for drug or alcohol problems alone. Unlike certain states in the USA there is no provision for controlling patients money or direct where they live to help treat their addiction.

Risk management in mental health also requires psychiatrists to remain involved with their patients and not to disengage on handing them over to an addiction service.

Any unitary programme that is meant to meet the needs for these patients would have to address these issues and blend risk management from mental health with that of addiction. Whilst not impossible this involves major adjustments in attitudes and raises concerns about areas of responsibility.

Prejudice and stigma

A patient with dual diagnosis raises prejudice from all sides. Attitudes about addiction being "self inflicted" and mental illness renders these individuals dangerous and unpredictable. The allocation of time and resource to their care may attract criticism not based in evidence, and hinders service development.

■ A wider picture of training research and development

Whilst the needs of the individual patient also need to be addressed there is also need for development and planning and research and coordination around this group of patients which is particularly difficult to do when they fall across so many stalls and between different philosophises and cultures. There is also a need for education of the workers who are seeing these patients and empowerment to deal with their problems. From a local survey in Haringey and data from Birmingham (ref COMPASS) we found there was an enormous need for further education and support around this area and the majority of people working in general psychiatry felt quite unskilled in addiction. Likewise in the addiction services generic workers reported that they did not feel they had the knowledge to differentiate psychiatric conditions. Indeed there is a mutual lack of understanding of what the referral points and contact points are in the system.

■ Solutions

For the financial and political reasons listed above we are not going to be able to achieve the integrated Dual Diagnosis programmes of the USA which take patients in for a period of several years are able to provide their social, housing and health care needs and have the funding attached to it. However the patients do exist and Dual Diagnosis is being addressed in the UK in a number of innovative systems.

Single designated expert worker

In the UK there a number of single worker systems being set up where workers are given the lead responsibility for Dual Diagnosis and are placed either in Community Mental Health Teams (CMHTs) or in addiction and are then required to both carry a case load and develop their colleagues expertise in this area. The supervision of these workers may be through mental health in some places in others its based in addiction services. These workers face a number of challenges including that of chronic overload of caseload also isolation and also of demoralisation in the face of the enormous needs of the Dual Diagnosis population they are trying to deal with. They may also be demoralised by the apparent difficulties of trying to integrate the systems that are very different, much in the same way, as the patients have tried to negotiate it and found it difficult.

Haringey dual Team Model

In my own locality in response to this difficulty the solution has been to raise a specialised team for Dual Diagnosis. This community team works in collaboration with mental health and substance misuse see diagram.

It is about broadening the spectrum of agencies involved with the patient and helping them to coordinate and deliver care as needed on a patient centered basis. It involves bridging gaps and advocating with the patients for access to resources (e.g. day hospital, work experience, etc). Essentially we have a core of workers who have expertise in both drugs alcohol and mental health and that any one interview with any one patient can draw upon this depth of skill. This is backed by Consultant Psychiatric time and good links to "donating" core services. The provision of the service to general adult psychiatry seems to provide the clinicians with security and a sense that they have explored the possibilities when dealing with very difficult and potentially disruptive patients.

The challenge for such a service in pulling together both resources in terms funding and staff and maintaining that in the face of prejudice and stigma is quite significant. There is a sense in which these patients require a lot of resource and if that concentrated into one place it may be seen as a target for cuts, budgetary restrictions, which may cast a shadow over the future.

> **The Haringey Dual Diagnosis Service**
>
> A newly funded, consultant led multi-disciplinary service, which functions along a model of addiction liaison into mental health. The service offers tiered interventions based on a comprehensive assessment including:
> - re-evaluation of mental health symptoms in the light of addictive behaviour;
> - short term interventions focused around harm minimisation;
> - longer term work along the lines of assertive outreach but addressing substance misuse issues.
>
> The service is also able to offer psychiatric style liaison into addiction services and *to facilitate the movement of patients* between addiction services and mental health services together with the *sharing of information and expertise across these boundaries and developing training for both groups of staff*. The service does not "take over from mental health" but *works in collaboration* with other professionals. The service is focused on people with severe mental health problems and substance misuse issues. Patients with personality disorder are not excluded as long as they are in contact with mental health services.

What do we do?

Services offered to patients

Assessment

It became apparent that a major part of the role of the team is to provide an accurate and detailed assessment. We use a multidisciplinary approach, which may take more than one appointment. The inclusion of time lines and standardized assessment tools (borrowed from both mental health and addiction even though they have not been formally tested in this group) all aid the aim of a clear summary of the current situation and background. We recognize that in the UK hospitals code diagnosis in ICD 10 but find that at assessment DSM IV may be a more helpful tool.

All referrals are allocated at the weekly multidisciplinary team meeting and assessments fed back the week of their completion. A written summary of the assessment is sent to the referrer with a management plan attached. (Note; High levels of written communications are essential to this team, needing significant levels of administrative support telephone lines and computer access. We often send multiple copies of letters to the consultant referrer, GP, Community Mental Health Team at a different address to the consultant, Hostel manager, etc. Patients have to give consent for information sharing unless there is an issue of risk when confidentiality may be breached, but we have found relatively few problems with this in practise.)

Assessments follow a bio psychosocial model and should include physical examination, routine blood tests and urine drug screening.

Short term interventions

The key to the model of service in Haringey [6] is the issue of it bridging gaps between other services to provide appropriate and as far as possible evidenced based treatment following the intensive diagnosis and assessment described above. Whilst the evidence base for interventions in "dual diagnosed" is limited the principles of interventions from psychiatry and addiction are followed. This requires a breadth of skills in the team from educational interventions to the obvious medical role of initiating medication such as antidepressants or methadone, to motivational interviewing, relapse prevention and psychotherapeutic skills as well as behavioural and social interventions such as liasing with housing and benefits agencies. We are aware that other services offer a specific intervention to the "dual diagnosed" patient (*e.g.* cognitive behavioural therapy) but when setting up our service we believed that the patients needed this flexibility and range with in one place. Indeed whilst the treatment systems battle with issues around provision for dual diagnosis the patients cross the boundaries with ease.

The aim of the short-term intervention is to do a focused, time limited piece of work and then pass the patient onto one of the long-term agencies (possibly having helped their staff to work more easily with this individual). This should in theory keep a through put with the team promoting a mix of case load and helping to protect against burn out and a service that is clogged and has an impossible waiting list. The time limit on these interventions is supposed to be twelve weeks, but in reality patients may over run or are re referred.

Assertive outreach

In conjunction with the assessment and short-term interventions the service has a limited number of places for on going assertive outreach. These 30 patients represent the more chronic psychiatric patients often with polysubstance abuse. They are taken on for a period of one year (renewable). These patients tend to have more unstable psychiatric illness and are more likely to be admitted under the mental health act than the group with short-term interventions. Their substance use tends to be multiple substances including alcohol and relatively few of them have needed substitute prescribing with methadone. The principles of the interventions with them tend to follow the evidence base from psychiatry.

Services offered to families

In parallel with the short-term interventions we also offer sessions for carers/family members. These focus on addiction education and support in coping with another persons drug problem.

Education and Teaching and Research

With the staff mix we have recruited we are aware that we have a significant amount of skill and expertise that can be shared both ways to addictions and mental health to the benefits of patients and staff. There is a rolling series of seminars planned but as part of the service evaluation we are seeking to establish a baseline about education and attitudes to allow review of our impact over time.

The issues and pressures surrounding research *versus* service provision will vary by location. In Haringey we are evaluating this service, but our main priority is the provision of clinical care.

All members of the team are involved in their own ongoing professional development, and attend and participate in conferences guideline development etc. Several people are doing or have completed higher degrees and we have found that a supportive attitud to study is a good antidote to the stresses of working with this group of patients and their complex problems.

Organisational Issues

As well as working directly with patients and staff there are areas in the organization the service is involved in. These include :

- confidentiality/sharing of information policy,
- drugs on ward policy (mental health),
- alcohol detoxification policy (mental health),
- "rough guide to addiction" on mental health wards,
- the service also attends local planning meetings in both Mental Health and addiction arenas.

Thus a fairly small clinical service tries to bridge the gaps that exist between addiction and mental health services in one borough of London [7]. The focus on clinical work rather than a research structure may be unusually at present, but reflects the experience of those involved in setting this up and the needs of the patients we see.

References

1. Abou-Saleh MT. Substance misuse and comorbid psychiatric disorders. *CPD Bulletin Psychiatry* 2000; 2: 61-7.
2. Drake RE, Bartels SJ, TeagueGB, Noordsy DL, Clarke RE. Treatment of in Substance abuse in Severely Mentally Ill Patients. *Journal of nervous and mental disorders* 1993; 181: 606-11.

3. Johnson S. Dual Diagnosis of severe mental illness and substance misuse: a case for specialist services? *British Journal of Psychiatry* 1997; 171: 205-8.
4. Mental Health Act 1983. HMSO.
5. Miller WR, Rollnick S. Motivational interviewing: Preparing people to change addictive behaviour. Guilford, New York, 1991.
6. OPCS Census data for London Borough of Haringey. Census. HMSO, 1991-1993.
7. Menezes PR, Johnson S, Thornicroft G, Marshall J, Prossor D, Bebbington P, Kuipers E. Drug and Alcohol Problems among Individuals with Severe Mental Illness in South London. *British Journal of Psychiatry* 1996; 168: 612-9.

Mentally ill substance abusers in Sweden. A 5-year follow-up of a multisite study of co-operation between psychiatric services and social authorities

A. Öjehagen, I. Schaar

Department of Clinical Neuroscience, Division of Psychiatry, University of Lund, Sweden

High rates of comorbidity between substance use disorders and other mental disorders have been shown both in epidemiological and clinical samples [1-4]. Among others Ziedonis and Dávanzo [5] underline that having both a psychiatric illness and a substance use disorder often implies great suffering and need of help in several areas, and outcome has been found to be less good in comparison to those with one disorder. The segregation of psychiatric and substance abuse treatment services has been found counterproductive with this population. Improvements have been reported from long-term follow-up studies of integrated treatment [6].

In Sweden, a mental health care reform took place on January 1st, 1995. The municipal social services were then given greater responsibility for patients who have a life-long psychiatric illness. Difficulties had been recognized in coordinating treatment and support between psychiatric health care and social services for those with concurrent psychiatric and substance abuse disorders. A multi-centre study was initiated by the Department of Social Affairs aimed at improving co-operation between the local services, psychiatric health care and social services, in the care of severely mentally ill substance abusers. Thereby improvement in substance use disorders, mental illness and their social situation would hopefully be facilitated. This study was followed-up after 1$^{1/2}$ years [7] and a new follow-up was then performed after 5 years.

The aim of the present paper is to present the main findings of the 5-year follow-up study.

■ Material and methods

In Sweden the Social Services have the main responsibility for services concerning treatment and prevention of substance use disorders, while detoxification occurs within the Health care system. There are also a few specialized clinics within the Health care system. Mental disorders are managed within psychiatric health care. During the past 10 years there has been a reduction of inpatient treatment. As concerns patients with both a substance use disorder and another mental disorder, there is lack of co-operation between psychiatric health services and social services.

Design of the study

Ten out of about 50 projects were included (n = 358 patients) representing both rural and urban settings and running over a period of three years (1995-1998). They were selected by The Swedish Board for Health and Welfare. The patients were known within the Psychiatric health care system and/or Social services as having both a substance use disorder and a severe mental disorder. The diagnoses before inclusion in the projects were performed by local psychiatrists, and the patients gave informed consent to take part in the investigations at start and at follow-up.

Among the ten projects, two models of co-operation were used. In four projects the treatment and support were administered by a special treatment team themselves, so called *treatment team*. The other six projects coordinated assessment and treatment planning in different ways and most of the support was delivered by ordinary services, so called *co-ordination team*.

The first evaluation was performed after $1^{1/2}$ years and a second follow-up after 5 years. At the 5-year follow-up eight projects participated with a follow-up interview.

The death rate was followed up after $1^{1/2}$ years and five years for all participants (n = 358).

Subjects

Initial characteristics are described in detail in an article by Schaar and Öjehagen [7]: The mean age was 40 ± 9 years, 66% were men, 15% were married/cohabiting, 15% were ordinarily employed and 78% had their own residence. As many as 62% of the patients had previously made at least one suicide attempt. They rated a low Quality of life [8].

Methods

Initially *psychiatric diagnoses* were made according to *DSM III-R*, *axis I*, *axis II* and *axis V* (the Global Assessment of Functioning Scale, GAF) [9]. The distribution of psychiatric diagnoses, axis I and axis II is presented in detail in a previous paper [7]. For a more general view of the profile of psychiatric disorders, four diagnostic subgroups were made according to the initial inclusion diagnostic criteria of severe mental illness:

Substance use disorders		Severe mental disorders	
Alcohol dep.	77%	Psychosis	28%
Illicit drugs	33%	Depression	18%
Legal drugs	13%	Borderline	24%
		Others	30%

The group "others" contains patients with other diagnoses, mostly anxiety disorders in combination with personality disorders. In all, 62% had a personality disorder, and 40% had both an axis I and an axis II diagnosis. Among illicit drugs: amphetamine dependence was the most common diagnosis, 21%, followed by cannabis, 10%, least common was use of opiates (2%). Eleven percent of the patients were dependent on tranquillizers and/or sedatives. In all 20% had more than one substance use disorder.

Other measurements used at start, after $1^{1/2}$ years and 5 years: The severity of substance abuse was evaluated by the *Addiction Severity Index* (ASI), a semi-structured interview providing sociodemographic information on both past and recent problems in seven areas of life functioning; medical status, employment and self-support, alcohol use, drug use, legal status, family and social relationships and psychiatric symptoms. A composite score is derived from each area, based exclusively on the last 30-day period, ranging from 0.0 = no problem to 1.0 = most severe problem [10, 11].

Psychological symptoms were estimated by the *Symptom Check List 90* (SCL-90), a self-report symptom inventory with 90-items on a 5-point scale of distress, from 0 = "not at all" to 4 = "extremely". The questions are scored and interpreted in terms of 9 primary symptom dimensions. These are labelled: somatization, obsessive-compulsive, interpersonal sensitivity, depression, anxiety, hostility, phobic anxiety, paranoid ideation and psychoticism. One of three global indices of distress is used in this presentation, the *Global Severity Index (GSI)* [12].

Quality of life (QoL), was measured by the use of Cantril's ladder [13], a global assessment included in the Lancashire life quality profile [14]. The patient estimates how life feels right now, lowest step 0 = terrible to highest step 100 = excellent [13]. At $1^{1/2}$ year and 5 years the following estimates were added, i.e. *The Clinical Rating scales (CRS) for Alcohol Use (AUS) and Drug Use (DUS)*, which have been developed for clinicians or case managers to assess and monitor substance use in persons with severe mental illness over time (in this study, the previous six months). Each of these scales estimates usage into one of five categories: abstinent, use without impairment, abuse, dependence and dependence with institutionalization [15].

Results

Follow-up after $1^{1/2}$ year

At the $1^{1/2}$ year follow-up 288 patients (84%) were interviewed. During the last 6 months before follow-up.

50% had no problems with alcohol/drugs (CRS), their psychological symptoms had decreased (GSI) and their Quality of life had improved. The social situation had stabilized, i.e. some had got a disability pension, while few so far had returned to work.

There were improvements in the severity of abuse according to the Composite score (ASI) in all areas except for employment [7].

Improvement according to different measurements was not related to sex, psychiatric diagnoses including substance abuse, or to co-operation models. Comparisons of improvements between the ten projects were not possible since they had different profiles as concerns mental disorders and substance abuse, some had more psychoses and some more drug abuse. The availability of services differed as well. Unfortunately we had no control group, i.e. with treatment and co-operation as usual.

Follow-up after 5 years

The mortality rate was increased:

0-3 yrs	14 (3.9%)
4-6 yrs	18 (5.0%)
All	32 (8.9%)

Causes of death were: suicide 3 people (0.8%), overdoses/intoxifications 12 people (3.4%), related to their abuse 13 (3.6%) and in 4 cases (1.1%) causes were unknown. A few initial characteristics were related to death, more men had died 11% (27/235) in comparison to women 4% (35/123), $p < .05$. More of those who had a personality disorder had died 12% (26/222) as compared to those who had no personality disorder 4% (6/136), $p < .05$.

Personal follow-up after 5 years

All but two projects took part in the 5-year follow-up. These two projects could not perform the follow-up interviews due to lack of financial support. Unfortunately we reached only 92 out of 221 patients who had been interviewed after $1^{1/2}$ year. Those 92 patients (42%) more often had a psychosis and alcohol dependence in comparison to those not interviewed initially. Seventy-four patients (33%) refused to participate. Initially they more often had a drug dependence and at the $1^{1/2}$ year follow-up they had a worse outcome as compared to those interviewed and those 55 (25%) who we could not reach for a follow-up interview. Some patients from the latter group had moved out of the region.

Among those who were interviewed, 23% had no alcohol consumption and 34% had a consumption level without a problem according to Clinical Rating Scale during the 6 months before follow-up. As concerns drugs, 68% had had no use of drugs.

Improvements in psychological symptoms (GSI), global functioning (GAF) and Quality of Life (QoL) are presented in *Figure 1*, giving the figures at start of the projects, after $1^{1/2}$ year and after 5 years. Improvement occurred during the project period, but there was no significant improvement thereafter. There were no differences between the projects (*Figure 1*).

Multisite study
5 years follow-up, interviewed (n=92)

	0 year		$1^{1/2}$ year		5 years
GSI	1.3 ± 0.7	***	1.0 ± 0.7	ns	1.0 ± 0.7
GAF	49 ± 11	***	57 ± 14	ns	59 ± 15
QoL	40 ± 27	***	58 ± 23	ns	61 ± 24

Figure 1. Psychological symptoms (GSI), global functioning (GAF) and Quality of Life (QoL) at start of the projects, after $1^{1/2}$ year and after 5 years (n = 92), Wilcoxon rank test: ** $P < 01$, * $P < .05$.

A comparison between ASI composite scores as measured initially, after $1^{1/2}$ year and after 5 years are presented in *Figure 2*. At $1^{1/2}$ year an improvement had occurred in alcohol, drug, and psychiatric problems. Between $1^{1/2}$ and 5 years improvements had occurred in legal matters and psychiatric problems (*Figure 2*).

The social situation at follow-up was as follows: 24% were married/cohabiting, 63% had a disability or were on long-term sick leave, and 80% had availability of an apartment or a flat.

Organisational level. After 5 years the projects stressed that in order to facilitate co-operation between psychiatric services and social services, there needed to be a decision to share the costs, which was the case in four of the projects after $1^{1/2}$ year. However, at the 5 year follow-up, coordinated care was planned on another three projects. Further they stressed it is of importance that a specialist staff, well educated in dual diagnoses, take care of these patients.

As concerns *treatment methods*, all projects stressed the need for an integration of treatments of both disorders. They drew attention to the use of structured methods, *i.e.* CBT (Cognitive Behavioural Therapy), DBT (Dialectic Behavioral Therapy), motivational strategies and the use of contracts including drug use control

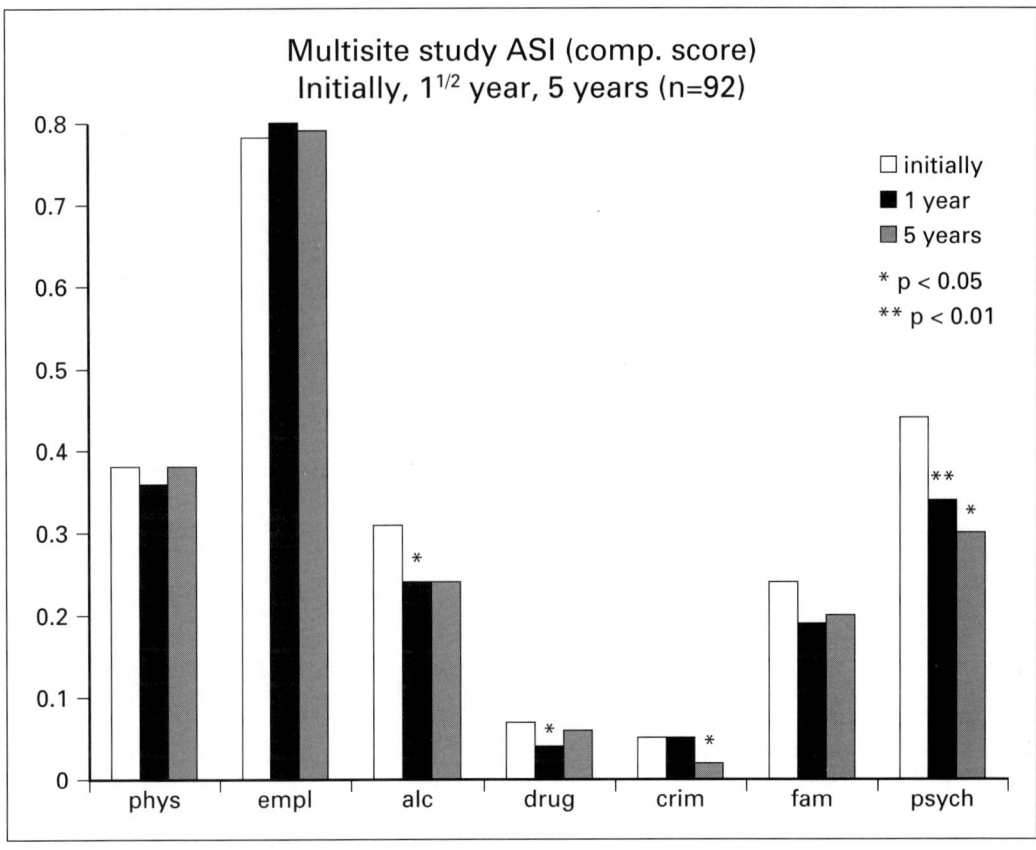

Figure 2. ASI composite scores, initially, after $1^{1/2}$ year and after 5 years; Wilcoxon rank test: ** $P < 01$, * $P < .05$.

■ Conclusion

The death rate is increased both in comparison to patients with a mental disorder and to patients who have only a substance use disorder. Certainly it is more difficult to treat patients who have both a substance use disorder and a severe mental illness. Therefore it is of importance to identify drug use and high consumption of alcohol early on. The positive effects of secondary intervention studies in patients with harmful use of alcohol (i.e. high consumtion) performed in primary health care have so far not been evaluated among psychiatric patients.

Among patients who could be interviewed, improvement occurred during the first $1^{1/2}$ year but not thereafter. The follow-up rate of patients who were interviewed was too low to make safe conclusions. There is further need for long-term follow-up studies on integrated treatment and support, and these preferably should be randomised controlled studies.

In Sweden the use of alcohol is increasing and illicit drugs are more available. Therefore national prevention plans are in place to meet the increasing use of alcohol and illicit drugs. Finally, The Swedish Council on Technology Assessment in Health Care (SBU) perform reviews of evidence-based methods used in health care. Such a review was published in 2001 as concerns treatment methods for alcohol and drug problems. A similar review concerning anxiety and mood disorders will probably be published in 2003.

References

1. Regier DA, Farmer ME, Rae DS, Locke BZ, Keith SJ, Judd LL, Goodwin FK. Comorbidity of Mental Disorder With Alcohol and Other Drug Abuse, Results from the Epidemiological Catchment Area (ECA) Study. JAMA 1990; 264 (19): 2511-8.
2. Kessler RC, McGonagle KA, Zhao S, Nelson CB, Hughes M, Eshleman Z, et al. Lifetime and 12-Month Prevalence of DSM-III-R Psychiatric Disorders in the United States. *Arch Gen Psychiatry* 1994; 51: 8-19.
3. Merikangas KR, Mehta RL, Molnar BE, Walters EE, Swendsen JD, Aguilar-Gaziola S, et al. Comorbidity Of Substance Use Disorders With Mood And Anxiety Disorders: Results Of The International Consortium. In Psychiatric Epidemiology. *Addictive Behaviors* 1998; 23 (6): 893-907.
4. Appleby L, Dyson V, Luchins D, Cohen L. The Impact of Substance Use Screening on a Public Psychiatric Inpatient Population. *Psychiatr Serv* 1997; 48 (10): 1311-6.
5. Ziedonis MD, Dávanzo K. *Schizoprenia and Substance Abuse*. Kranzler HJ, Rounsaville BJ, ed. *Dual Diagnosis and Treatment*. New York: Marcel Dekker, 1998: chapter 14.
6. Drake RE, Mercer-McFadden C, Mueser KT, McHugo GJ, Bod GR. Review of integrated mental health and substance abuse treatment for patients with dual diagnoses. *Schizophr Bull* 1998; 24: 589-608.
7. Schaar I, Öjehagen A. Severely mentally ill substance abusers: an 18-month follow-up study. SPPE, *Social Psychiatry and Psychiatric Epidemiology* 2001; 36 (2): 70-8.
8. Schaar I, Öjehagen A. Predictors of improvement in quality of life of severely mentally ill substance abusers during 18 months of co-operation between psychiatric and social services. SPPE, *Social Psychiatry and Psychiatric Epidemiology* 2002: 37.
9. American Psychiatric Association (1987). *Diagnostic and Statistical Manual of Mental Disorders*, 3rd edn, revised. American Psychiatric Association, Washington DC, 1987.
10. McLellan AT, Kusher H, Metzger D, Peters R, Smith I, Grissom G, et al. The fifth edition of the Addiction Severity Index: Historical critique and normative data. *Journal of Substance Abuse Treatment* 1992; 9: 199-213.
11. Bergman H, Andréasson S, Armélius BÅ, Berglund M, Larsson H, Rydberg U, Tengvald K. The translation of the ASI manual into Swedish language, CUS, 1996.
12. Derogatis LR. *Administration, Scoring & Procedures Manual-I*, for the Revised version. Psychometrics Research Unit, John Hopkins University Scool of Medicine, Baltimore, 1979.
13. Cantril H. *The Pattern of Human Concerns*. New Brunswick, NJ: Rutgers University Press, 1965.
14. Oliver J, Huxley P, Bridges K, Mohammed H. *Quality of life and mental health services*. London: Routledge, 1996.
15. Mueser KT, Drake RE, McHugo GJ, Mercer-McFadden C, Ackerson TH. Toolkit for Evaluating Substance Abuse in Persons with Severe Mental Illness. Evaluation Cernter HSRI, NewHampshire, USA, 1995.

Heroin assisted treatment of drug addicts

M. Krausz

Centre of Interdisciplinary Addiction Research/Universität Hamburg

---

Introduction of heroin assisted treatment for chronically addicted heroin users has been a much discussed topic since the beginning of the 1990s. Faced with the increase in drug related deaths and the spread of HIV-infections and AIDS among drug users, the city of Hamburg proposed a new law in May 1992 to change the BtMG, with the aim of enabling medical heroin treatment.

With the start of the Swiss project (PROVE) in 1994, the debate about the introduction of a German trial for heroin assisted treatment intensified. In the meantime, Germany had also acquired experience with the efficiency of methadone treatment. Knowledge about its possibilities and limitations had a great impact on the discussion of alternatives for heroin treatment. The German discussion reached a climax with the publication of the Swiss results in the summer of 1997 [1, 2], in which an altogether positive evaluation of the treatment was presented.

Presently, heroin may not be legally prescribed. According to the currently applicable [3] German narcotic law (BtMG) the use of heroin is only allowed in exceptional cases for scientific use or other important purposes that are in the public interest.

Heroin assisted treatment is to be targeted at heroin addicts that are in need of treatment and have not been able to make use of existing addiction treatment networks and those that failed to respond to existing treatments. Heroin assisted treatment should thus be understood as a controlled substitution with pure heroin in a *structured treatment setting*.

Beyond the clinical examination of the drug, special studies concerning criminology, the care system (health, economy, implementation, co-operation), cognitive-motor and neuropsychological questioning as well as internal evaluation of psychosocial care will be examined and integrated in a 24-month study.

■ Clinical traits

Heroin (3,6-diacetylmorphine) is a half synthetic opioid and is derived from morphine by acetylisation. The analgesic action lasts for about 4 to 5 hours, but the elimination half-life of the heroin itself amounts to only 3-9 minutes. 6-acetylmorphine and morphine are the active substances. Heroin was first synthesised in England in 1874, while commercial production started in 1898 by the German company Bayer. The medication was mainly used for pulmonary disorders and found wide distribution in times of tuberculosis. Unlike for morphine, the addiction potential was not described until the 1920s, which lead to an implementation of stricter controls for production and use of heroin.

Heroin has a strong analgesic effect, but also leads to nausea, dry mouth, and circulatory disorders. Other organic effects are a reduction in breathing frequency, reduced appetite and slowed colon function. Regular heroin consumption among women can lead to menstruation disorders including amenorrhea. Mental effects are manifold. The rapid flooding of the brain by heroin (unlike morphine) leads to a strong euphoric effect and intensive feeling of well-being, which can lead to a long-lasting state of sedation (trance).

The consumption of heroin has a high risk of leading to addiction. Longer lasting regular consumption can lead to withdrawal symptoms when discontinuing heroin, with cold-like symptoms such as the flu, increased flow of tears, muscular pains, fever and sleep disorders as well as a feeling of unrest, irritability and general discomfort, lasting for about one week.

■ Background for heroin assisted treatment in Germany

In Germany there are currently about 150,000 *heroin addicts*. Approximately 35% to 40% of these receive maintenance treatment, predominately with methadone. About 700 drug addicts are presently in abstinence oriented out-patient rehabilitation and nearly 10,000 in in-patient detoxification programmes [4].

The dangers of untreated opiate addiction on an individual and social level are extremely high. Especially older addicts who are not in adequate treatment have an increased mortality risk [5, 6] and are likely to suffer from chronic illness such as hepatitis, HIV/AIDS and other infections. Often their living circumstances are marked by social marginalisation. Among those undergoing methadone treatment, the mortality rate is substantially higher when therapy is unsuccessful than when the addicts are successfully treated [6]. On a social level, opiate addiction is the cause of significant costs in the form of crime and the treatment of accompanying illnesses [7, 8]. The (regional) burdens from open drug scenes are severe, especially in big cities [9, 10].

When considering a rather conservative estimate of 35,000 methadone-maintained and at least 35,000 currently untreated opiate addicts, the number of potentially suited patients for a heroin assisted treatment in Germany can be estimated to be at least 3,500 to 7,000 of those maintained (corresponding to 10%-20%) and another approximately 10,000 (30%) of the untreated group.

Heroin assisted treatment seems to arise from the limitations of the present system of care which fails to adequately reach a certain proportion of addicts – that do not come, that do not stay or where treatment does not show any substantial results. Heroin treatment is considered the *"ultimo ratio"*, thus it should be considered as an addition to the current addiction care system. The primary goal of treatment remains abstinence or maintenance, as in previous treatment forms.

■ International experiences

Experience with the prescription of heroin to drug addicts has been accumulated in Great Britain and Switzerland. The Netherlands have also been running a clinical study in 6 cities, since mid 1998.

Great Britain

Since 1920 it has been possible to prescribe heroin in special clinics throughout Great Britain. The best known British study by Hartnoll *et al.* [11], a randomized comparison between heroin and methadone patients, showed no clear preference for or against either treatment. Results showed that the abstinence rate among methadone treated patients after one year was higher while those treated with heroin had a significantly lower drop-out rate. A study by Battersby *et al.* [12] with 40 patients, who were prescribed injected methadone or heroin, failed to reach a conclusion about the efficacy and importance of these therapies. About a third of the participants showed some improvement, however the social conditions of eight patients had considerably deteriorated (20%) towards the end of their treatment (after an average of 45 weeks). A further study originates from the largest heroin prescription clinic in west London. 58 patients that were given the choice between heroin and methadone were included in the study. 37 decided to inject heroin. The remaining 21 injected methadone [13, 14]. After three months 50 patients (86%) had remained in treatment and after 12 months the number had reduced to 33 (57%). Among those that remained in treatment, there was a substantial decrease in the consumption of illicit drugs and the associated risk behaviour as well as a decline in criminal activities. Further, there was an improvement in general health and social integration. Unfortunately there was no comparison made between the heroin and methadone groups.

Switzerland

In 1994 Switzerland launched the "The Medical Prescription of Narcotics Research Programme" (PROVE). 1,146 patients in total participated. The project was conducted in 18 centres in 15 cities. The collection of data was completed in 1996. There are currently two interim reports and one final report [1, 2]. Further reports concerning the special analyses will follow. Unlike the British studies, the Swiss were able to conclude with a clear recommendation, for the continuation of a restricted, and target group oriented heroin assisted treatment in special clinics. Furthermore, they were able to show that such a project can be realised. The retention rate was relatively high at 89% after 6 months and 69% after 18 months. The positive effects of heroin prescription were demonstrated in regard to development of health, social integration and especially in a dramatic decrease in criminal activities. The consumption of (illicit) heroin and cocaine showed a distinct and rapid decrease, while consumption of alcohol and cannabis remained virtually the same.

As part of the Swiss project, they carried out a randomized control group study comparing heroin patients to patients in other types of treatment [15]. A group of patients that had been selected according to the Swiss indication criteria for heroin addiction, were randomly assigned either to heroin assisted treatment or to a six months waiting list. During the waiting time they had the possibility to receive another type of medical treatment. After the six months period the second group was given the possibility to take part in the heroin assisted treatment. Originally the aim had been to have approximately 40 patients in each group, however only 73 people showed an interest to take part in the study. Of these 73 only 57 fulfilled the requirements set by the study. After the six months period they had results for 27 heroin patients and 21 from the control group, most of which had started a methadone treatment. Heroin patients showed a significant decrease in the consumption of illicit heroin and benzodiazepines. Furthermore, there was a decrease in suicide attempts in comparison to the control group where an increase was observed. In the heroin group, a greater number received medical treatment for their mental problems. Finally, the experimental group showed a marked decrease in illegal income connected with a decrease in criminal indictments.

Netherlands

In July 1998 the Netherlands started a project for medical co-prescription of heroin for long-term heroin addicts. Pilot studies in Amsterdam and Rotterdam failed to yield any procedural problems, and the project was extended to the cities of The Hague, Groningen, Heerlen/Maastricht and Utrecht in 1999, as originally planned [16]. Only methadone maintained patients were accepted for treatment [17]. Furthermore, inhaled as well as injected heroin was offered in an attempt to integrate the fact that in the Netherlands the predominant form of consumption for heroin is smoking.

The heroin prescription project has been carried out as a clinical study according to the standards of "Good Clinical Practice". The aim of the study is to evaluate the efficacy of a combined methadone-heroin treatment across a period of 12 months in comparison to a 12 months oral methadone treatment in regard to the reduction of illicit drug consumption as well as an improvement of the health status and the social integration of chronic, treatment resistant heroin addicts [18]. In the three fold experimental design, in which the injected and inhaled heroin are separately assessed, (study period of 20 months) the randomized experimental groups A, B and C were given heroin, in addition to the methadone they received, at varying time intervals. After a two months preparation phase, that served as a period of clarification of indication and willingness for treatment, group B (N = 115) received heroin in addition to methadone for a 12 month period, while group A (N = 135) received methadone only. After completion of this initial phase, group A – as a form of motivation to remain in the control group for the rest of the study – was prescribed heroin for 6 months. Group B received no heroin and was treated with methadone (for another 6 months). The experimental group C (N = 125) was also prescribed heroin, however in contrast to group B, this group received this for six months after the initial six months (following the randomisation period) when members were exclusively maintained on methadone. This structure enables analyses of differing efficacy between a 6- and 12-month heroin treatment.

Primary outcome criteria was a minimum 40% improvement of state of health or social integration. Illicit drug consumption – in this case cocaine – should not rise above 20%. The thus defined response has to differ by more than 20% after 12 months between the heroin group (b) and the 12 months methadone group (A). In a further multivariate assessment, a number of secondary analyses are planned, to investigate the possible association of patient and setting variables to the outcome criteria.

In May 1999, 187 patients were randomly assigned to one of two groups, 115 to the inhalation group and 72 to the injection group. The participation rate for the 2 months collection and investigation is currently at about 82%. With completion of the first project phase in Amsterdam and Rotterdam, there were no noteworthy problems concerning recruitment, randomisation and data collection. Furthermore, there were no medical emergencies and no problems with public acceptance of the heroin treatment.

The report was presented in the beginning of 2002 and could show that heroin assisted treatment was able to improve the health of the target group. It was feasible and effective.

■ Tentative conclusions

All these studies and observations have in common that heroin assisted treatment is possible and also accepted [19]. The British studies are inconclusive as to whether the use of heroin has merits justifying significant extra costs or problems, but seems to prove that its use is feasible and might have benefits for some patients. The Swissprojects further demonstrate that heroin treatment seems to increase the therapeutic potential insofar as groups not benefiting from methadone maintenance are attracted to heroin prescription projects. Further, the treatment improves health and social functioning in these treatment resistant patients. The existence of heroin projects seems not to decrease motivation for other types of treatment. The Dutch projects strongly indicate that patients not making progress in methadone maintenance will benefit if offered an additional treatment of heroin. If the additional treatment is stopped, the patients will lose their progress.

Obviously, the research at present can prove that the use of heroin within structured therapeutic settings might benefit patients, in particular seemingly treatment resistant subject. As Gossop [20] points out, some of the features might be connected to the strict rules connected to heroin prescription with attendance three times a day and no take-home dosages. This actualises the question of capacity and resources in the treatment system. Nevertheless, present research indicates that use of heroin might benefit individuals in severe states of addiction. Further research is needed to broaden our knowledge. The German position is that heroin assisted treatment would justify itself if the results of research confirm that the desired (individual) effects cannot be reached with currently established therapies. This question is to be analysed in an ongoing German model project for heroin assisted treatment, in which the treatment results are to be compared with a control group of methadone treated subjects.

References

1. Uchtenhagen A, Gutzwiller F, Dobler-Mikola A. Versuche für eine ärztliche Verschreibung von Betäubungsmitteln. Abschlußbericht der Forschungsbeauftragten. Synthesebericht. Zürich, 1997.
2. Uchtenhagen A, Dobler-Mikola A, Steffen T, Gutzwiller F, Blättler R, Pfeifer S. *Prescription of Narcotics for Heroin Addicts. Main Results of the Swiss National Cohort Study*. In: Uchtenhagen A, Gutzwiller F, Dobler-Mikola A, Steffen T, Rihs-Middel M, eds. *Medical Precription of Narcotics*, Vol. 1. Basel: Karger, 1999.
3. Gölz J. Methadonsubstitution in der Arztpraxis. In: Gölz J (Hrsg.). Der drogenabhängige Patient. 2. Aufl. München: Urban & Fischer; 1999; S. 282-312.

4. Holz A, Leune J. Versorgung Suchtkranker in Deutschland. In: DHS (Hrsg.). Jahrbuch Sucht '99. Geesthacht: Neuland; 1998; S. 154-74.
5. Grönbladh L, Öhlund LS, Gunne LM. Mortality in heroin addiction: impact of methadone treatment. *Acta Psychiatrica Scandinavica* 1990; 82: 223-7.
6. Raschke P, Püschel K, Heinemann A. Raschgiftmortalität und Substitutionstherapie in Hamburg (1990-1998). *Suchttherapie* 2000; 1: 43-8.
7. Hartwig KH, Pies I. Rationale Drogenpolitik in der Demokratie. Tübingen: JCB Mohr, 1995.
8. Bathsteen M, Legge I, Rabitz-Suhr S. *Delinquenz polizeibekannter KonsumentInnen harter Drogen*. In: Krausz M, Raschke P (Hrsg.). Drogen in der Metropole. Freiburg: Lambertus; 1999; S. 111-26.
9. Renn H, Lange KJ. Stadtviertel und Drogenszene. Eine vergleichende Untersuchung zur Belästigung durch "offene" Drogenszenen in europäischen Großstädten. Hamburg, 1995.
10. Homann B, Paul B, Thiel G, Wams M. Drogenkonsum und Gesundheitsraumbedarf in der Hamburger "offenen Drogenszene". *Sucht* 2000; 46: 129-36.
11. Hartnoll RL, Mitcheson MC, Battersby A, Brown G, Ellis M, Fleming P, Hedley N. Evaluation of heroin maintenance in controlled trial. *Arch Gen Psychiatry* 1980; 37 (8): 877-84.
12. Battersby M, Strang J, Farrell M, Gossop M, Robson P. "Horsetrading": Prescribing injectable opiates to opiate addicts – a descriptive study. *Drug & Alcohol Review* 1992; 11: 35-42.
13. Metrebian N, Shanahan W, Stimson GV. Heroin prescribing in the United Kingdom. *European Addiction Research* 1996; 2: 194-200.
14. Metrebian N, Shanahan W, Wells B, Stimson GV. Feasibility of prescribing injectable heroin and methadone to opiate-dependent drug users: associated health gains and harm reductions. *The Medical Journal of Australia* 1998; 168: 596-600.
15. Perneger TV, Giner F, del Rio M, Mino A. Randomised trial of heroin maintenance programme for addicts who fail in conventional drug treatments. *British Medical Journal* 1998; 317: 13-8.
16. Central Committee on the Treatment of Heroin Addicts CCBH (1997 a) Investigating the medical prescription of heroin. Utrecht.
17. Central Committee on the Treatment of Heroin Addicts CCBH (1997 b) A randomized clinical study to evaluate, in chronic treatment-refractory heroin addiction, the effectiveness of a new treatment regimen, medically co-prescribed heroin and oral methadone compared to the standard treatment oral methadone alone. Reference Document.
18. van den Brink W, Hendriks VM, van Ree JM. Medical co-prescription of heroin to chronic, treatment-resistant methadone patients in the Netherlands. *Journal of Drug Issues* 1999; 29: 587-607.
19. Krausz M, Uchtenhagen A, van den Brink W. Medizinisch indizierte Heroinverschreibung in der Behandlung Drogenabhängiger. Klinische Versuche und Stand der Forschung in Europa. *Sucht* 1999; 45: 171-86.
20. Gossop M. The Dutch Heroin Trial: Issues and Implications. *Sucht* 2002; 48: 304-6.

Treatment system and intervention strategies for mentally ill substance abusers: the Greek experience

K. Nicolaou

Specialist Psychiatrist Dependency Unit 18 Ano, Psychiatric Hospital of Attica, Leoforos Athinon, Dafni, Athens, Greece

Services in Greece are advanced, long-term programmes offering high-quality treatment but limited to the large rural areas, inadequate to cover the actual number of users. This discrepancy reflects the lack of a coordinated national policy.

Dual diagnosis patients are the least resourced group of patients within psychiatric services, and Greece is no exception, faced with stigmatisation and discrimination. Polarity of services and rejection of care providers is often the case.

The only specialised Dual Diagnosis Unit in the country is part of the Dependency Department 18 Ano of the Psychiatric Hospital of Attica in Athens.

The majority of dual diagnosis patients presenting with less severe disorders are accepted to the residential stage of the programme. Severe mental disorders (schizophrenia or other psychosis, bipolar disorder, severe personality disorder) are referred to the special out-patient Unit which functions as a day-centre providing psychiatric care, supportive group – and individual psycho-therapy, art – and drama-therapy, family therapy. The programme extends over years with practically no time limit and relapses in substance use are tolerated. Patients are usually hospitalized, when needed, in a general psychiatric ward under the unit's supervision.

About 50-70% complete the second phase (the residential stage). Follow-up for 9 months during rehabilitation shows a relapse rate of about 20%. Dual diagnosis patients show a higher drop-out rate. About 10-12% of all patients are referred to the Dual Diagnosis Unit. Retention rates seem quite promising, data are currently under examination.

An effective national policy should also address this group of patients. Less severe cases, which are the majority, should be managed in conventional drug-services with little adjustment of the services' context and specialized programmes should be limited to severe cases.

■ The situation in Greece

The Greek public and the Greek scientific community were very disillusioned in the late eighties to realise that traditional social structure and strong family ties wouldn't prevent a western type drug epidemic. The indicators of drug use are still increasing steadily reaching the numbers of other European countries with an at least ten years' delay. Other European countries are already showing a stabilisation or even a decrease as a result of planning and introducing a nationwide policy [1]. The new trends in substance use are now similar to other countries with some cultural differences. A lot has been done ever-since in terms of reduction in demand and availability but I'm afraid there's still no national strategy with a definite action-plan and long-term goals [1]. On the other hand almost all existing services are advanced, long-term programmes offering high-quality treatment services at all levels but limited to the large rural areas and not enough to meet all users either in number or in special needs. This discrepancy reflects the lack of a coordinated national policy.

The attitude and expectations of both users and staff in Greece have been determined by the two largest drug-organisations in the country that both follow the principles of the therapeutic communities and date back to the early eighties. Concepts like harm-reduction and maintenance with substitutes have been introduced with some difficulty and treatment remains largely synonymous with abstinence. There are practically no services providing in-patient Detoxification. Substitution programmes are abstinence-oriented as well (long-term detoxification or maintenance with subsequent rehabilitation) with strict on site dispensing, resulting in long waiting lists. A recent attempt in the opposite direction is Buprenorphine dispension in general psychiatric units. Substitution Programmes are under the direct control of the Organisation against Drugs, OKANA, which is assigned by the Ministry of Health the planning, promotion and co-ordination of a national policy [1].

Co-morbidity

The co-morbidity of substance use and mental illness has been recognized for years but the real dimensions of both the prevalence [2-5] and the problems associated with this group of patients haven't been acknowledged until fairly recently.

The other most common diagnosis among substance users is misusing another substance followed by personality disorders and depression. Severe mental illness (schizophrenia or other psychosis, bipolar disorder) may be less common, shows however a much greater impact on the individual (course, prognosis, psychopathology and management, suicide risk, compliance and treatment, social consequences like homelessness) [6-11], on society (criminality- and violence issues) [12] and on the health system (higher treatment costs) [13, 14].

This group of patients is the least resourced within psychiatric services, and Greece is no exception, faced with stigmatisation and discrimination. Polarity of services and rejection of care providers is often the case. General psychiatric services are usually unwilling and reluctant to deal with the substance related problems of the patient. The diagnosis of drug-induced psychosis [15], their antisocial behaviour and non-compliance are usually the excuse for refusing admission or an early discharge [16]. On the other hand specialized alcohol and drug programmes are often too confrontative and stressful for the psychotic patient, with strict limits on abstinence and a suspiciousness on behalf of the staff about taking even prescribed medication. This reflects in both cases lack of training, experience and confidence of the staff, inability and inadequacy of the services to deal with these complicated patients [17]. The result is that they are usually undertreated or "receive no treatment at all" [18]. A joined attempt of both services may end up in a "fragmentation" and a diffusion of responsibility that could have a negative effect on maintaining commitment and establishing relationships in an already non-compliant group [17, 18].

Dual-diagnosis programmes in Greece

Substitution Programmes in Greece do accept dual diagnosis patients and there is psychiatric care available but not a specialised programme. As long as they may be managed within the context of the programmes they do remain on. They are otherwise referred to general psychiatric units or to the only available specialized programme for dual diagnosis patients in Greece, which is part of one of these large drug services. The Athens University Clinic has one outpatient-Unit for Substance Use and they accept uncomplicated cases as well. All other services refer everybody in need of psychiatric attention and medication to this very same unit (*Figure 1*).

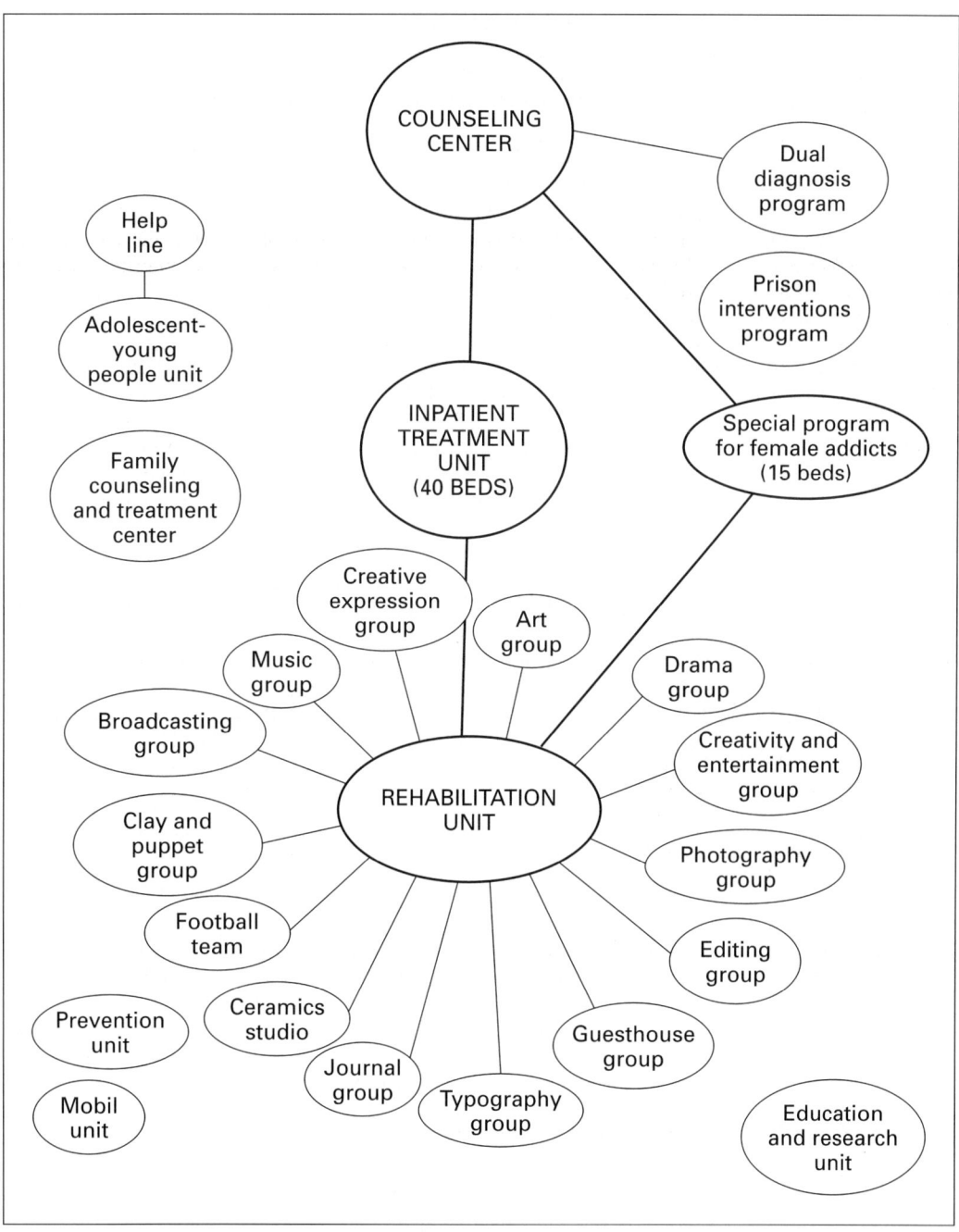

Figure 1.

The Dependency Department 18 Ano of the Psychiatric Hospital of Attica in Athens, technically an NHS-Clinic on the premises of a psychiatric hospital is a "luxurious" programme lasting over 18 months directing drug users through different stages of therapy including six months in a therapeutic community and nine months rehabilitation and follow-up (actually involving education, training and social rehabilitation).

The department includes various units, community based and in-patient clinics and covers a very broad range of patients' needs. These services address special groups such as Women, Women with children, Teenagers, Families, Prison Population, Alcoholics and Dual Diagnosis patients. About 500 drug users are attended at all units of the department on a single day by a multi-disciplinary team.

The Department follows the therapeutic-continuum concept, *i.e.* a client is followed-up from day one at the Counseling service all the way through to Rehabilitation via a closed Therapeutic Community attended by the same therapist all along. The treatment model involves intensive, client-centered, insight-orientated group – and individual psychotherapy, art – and drama-therapy, occupational therapy, coping skills and relapse prevention techniques. No substitutes are given. Detoxification is achieved on an outpatient basis with pharmacological help.

All clients are thoroughly assessed at the initial phase at the Counseling service. An ego structure along with interpersonal and cognitive skills that enable the patients to cope with the psychotherapy processes are a precondition for entering the second phase of the programme in the therapeutic community.

The majority of dual diagnosis patients presenting with less severe disorders such as personality disorders, depression or anxiety disorders are accepted to the second phase together with other drug users. Constant psychiatric care, medication and individualized approach are provided. They otherwise have to follow all of the community's activities. Suicidal patients or patients presenting with self-destructive actions or even psychotic symptoms have been accepted at times as long as they were able to follow the community's curriculum.

Severe mental disorders (schizophrenia or other psychosis, bipolar disorder, severe personality disorder such as border-line) are referred to the special out-patient Unit which functions as a day-centre accessible for 10 hours a day, providing psychiatric care, supportive group – and individual psychotherapy, art – and drama-therapy, family therapy. It is an integrated treatment model taking in consideration various needs of the patients, the goal is stabilisation. The programme extends over years (there is practically no time limit) and relapses in substance use are tolerated. Therapeutic interventions are introduced according to each patient's mental condition and readiness to change. The multi-disciplinary team may take care of about 20 patients a day and is very careful in creating an empathic, safe and warm atmosphere.

Hospitalisation of psychiatric relapses is an unresolved matter usually dealt on a personal basis, an arrangement between psychiatrists. Patients are hospitalised in a general psychiatric ward under the unit's supervision.

Continuity of care, providing integrated programmes of treatment, trying to meet all patients' needs in the same setting means managing and changing the risk factors, stabilizing and improving the mental disorders and reducing the hazardous complications.

■ Outline of an integrated model service

An ideal service would have to provide *(table I)*, in addition to what I have already said: a 24 hour access, coverage of immediate needs such as accommodation, food, financial and legal problems and an in-patient clinic for hospitalization when needed.

Prototype services like this are the "continuous treatment teams" established in New Hampshire community mental health centres by Robert Drake [17-19].

Table I. Outline of an integrated model service.

Meet all the patients' needs in the same setting

- easily accessible
- capability to meet immediate needs (accommodation, food, legal and financial problems)
- psychiatric care
- supportive group- and individual- psychotherapy
- long-term stage-wise interventions
- training in coping-skills and relapse prevention
- art- and drama-therapy
- relapses in substance use are tolerated
- possibility of hospitalisation when needed
- family involvement
- no time-limit
- social rehabilitation

Effectiveness

Substitution Programmes in Greece show a completion rate slightly higher than the european average [20]. Therapeutic communities show similar results to international standards [21]. In our programme about 50-70% complete the second phase (the residential stage). Follow-up for 9 months during rehabilitation shows a relapse rate of about 20%. There's no longer follow-up. Dual diagnosis patients show a higher drop-out rate. There's a study going on to determine differences in retention rates and drop-out rates according to psychopathology.

About 10-12% of all patients are referred to the Dual Diagnosis Unit. Retention rates seem quite promising but more systematic examination of the data is needed since some patients interrupt for months or even years, some have an irregular and some a systematic attendance, and indicators such as number of relapses in substance use and number of hospitalizations should also be taken in account.

Conclusion

The Organisation against Drugs (Okana) has designed, last year, a 5-year action-plan involving all levels of demand reduction. An effective national policy should also address this group of patients: more drug services all over the country, specialised units, education of general psychiatric and drug-services staff, liaison of services with each other in order to improve their respective competence [22]. Less severe cases, which are the majority, should be managed in conventional drug-services with little adjustment of the services' context and specialised programmes should be limited to severe cases. Continuity of care, providing integrated programmes of treatment, trying to meet all patients' needs in the same setting means managing and changing the risk factors, stabilizing and improving the mental disorders and reducing the hazardous complications.

References

1. Greek Focal Point Of Emcdda. *Annual Report on Greece* 2000.
2. Marsden J, Gossop M, Stewart D, Rolfe A, Farrell M. Psychiatric symptoms among clients seeking treatment for drug dependence. Intake from the National Treatment Outcome Research Study. *British Journal of Psychiatry* 1996; 176: 285-9.
3. Menezez PR, Johnson S, Thornicroft G, et al. Drug and alcohol problems among individuals with severe mental problems in South London. *British Journal of Psychiatry* 1996; 169: 334-7.
4. Soyka M, Albus M, Kathmann N, et al. Prevalence of alcohol and drug abuse in schizophrenic inpatients. *European archives of Psychiatry and Clinical Neuroscience* 1993; 242: 362-72.

5. Regier DA, Farmer ME, Rae DS, et al. Comorbidity of mental disorders with alcohol and other drug abuse: Results from the Epidemiologic Catchment area (ECA) Study. *Journal of American Mental Association* 1990; 264 (9): 2511-8.
6. Feinmann JA, Dunner DL. The effect of alcohol and substance abuse on the course of bipolar affective disorder. *Journal of affective disorders* 1996; 37 (1): 43-9.
7. Krausz M, Massr, Haasen C, Gross J. Psychopathology in patients with schizophrenia and substance abuse. *Psychopathology* 1996; 29: 95-103.
8. Owen RR, Fischer ER, Booth BM. Medication, non-compliance and substance abuse Among patients with schizophrenia. *Psychiatric Services* 1996; 47 (8): 853-8.
9. Brady KT, Sonne SC. The relationship between substance abuse and bipolar disorder. *Journal of Clinical Psychiatry* 1995; 56 (suppl 3): 19-24.
10. D'mello DA, Boltz MK, Msibi B. Relationship between concurrent substance abuse in psychiatric patients and neuroleptic dosage. *American Journal of Drug and Alcohol Abuse* 1995; 21 (2): 257-65.
11. Arndt S, Tyrrell G, Flaum M. Comorbidity of substance abuse and schizophrenia: the role of premorbid adjustment. *Psychological Medicine* 1992; 22: 379-88.
12. Johns A. Substance misuse: a primary risk and a major problem of comorbidity. *International Review of Psychiatry* 1997; 9: 233-41.
13. Haywood TW, Krawitz HM, Grossman LS, et al. Predicting the "revolving door" phenomenon among patients with schizophrenic, schizoaffective and affective disorders. *American Journal of Psychiatry* 1995; 152 (6): 856-61.
14. Bartels SJ, Teague GB, Drake RE. Substance abuse in schizophrenia: service utilization and costs. *Journal of Nervous and Mental Disease* 1993; 181: 227-32.
15. Gunn J. Personality disorders and forensic Psychiatry. *Clinical Behaviour and Mental Health* 1992; 2: 202-11.
16. Fariello D, Scheidt S. Clinical case management of the dually diagnosed patient. *Hospital and Community Psychiatry* 1989; 40: 1065-7.
17. Johnson S. Dual diagnosis of severe mental illness and substance misuse: a case for specialist services? *British Journal of Psychiatry* 1997; 171: 205-8.
18. Smith J, Hucker S. Schizophrenia and substance abuse. *British Journal of Psychiatry* 1994; 165: 13-21.
19. Drake RE. Substance use reduction among patients with severe mental illness. *Community Mental Health Journal* 1996; 32 (3): 311-4.
20. Tsaklakidou D, Douzenis A, Malliori M, Okana. Treatment results of the first 211 admissions to the Substitution Unit of Athens. Announcement at the "World Psychiatric Congress". Regional Congress of preventive Psychiatry, 24-28 February 1999, Athens, Greece.
21. Kethea. Assessment of the Effectiveness of the Kethea-Therapeutic Communities, 2001.
22. Uchtenhagen A. ITACA/ADAT International Seminar: Drug Addiction Treatment and Care: "Services responding to clients' needs or clients adapting to organization or services?" (Personal Communication, 2000).

Dialectical behavior therapy of borderline patients with and without substance use problems: implementation and long term effects*

L. M.C. van den Bosch[1], R. Verheul[2], G. M. Schippers[3], Wim Van Den Brink[3]

1. Amsterdam Institute for Addiction Research, University of Amsterdam
2. Department of Clinical Psychology, University of Amsterdam, Psychotherapy Institute "Viersprong", Halsteren
3. Amsterdam Institute for Addiction Research, University of Amsterdam

---

Borderline personality disorder (BPD) is a persistent and severe mental disorder. Studies have shown significant co-morbidity between borderline personality disorder (BPD) and substance use disorders (SUD) or substance abuse (SA) [1-8]. The reported prevalence rates of SUD among patients with BPD range from 39% to 84% with a median rate of 67% [2, 9-11]. Within substance abuse populations, the prevalence of BPD ranges from 2% to 66% with a median rate of 18% [12]. Co-morbidity of SUD and BPD can partly be accounted for by overlapping diagnostic criteria [4, 13], but prevalence rates of BPD remain high even when substance abuse is excluded as a diagnostic criterion of BPD [4, 13]. Some have suggested that SUD and BPD are causally linked in some way [14]. For example, some have hypothesized that SUD and BPD may share a common aetiology and may be viewed best as being in the same domain of psychopathology, *i.e.*, affective dysregulation [15, 16] or impulse control disorders [11, 17]. Many authors view substance use as a manifestation of impulsivity which is a core feature of borderline personality disorder [18, 19].

Since substance abuse can be considered a typical borderline manifestation rather than an independent comorbid condition, it is interesting that borderline patients comorbid with substance abuse (SA) often are treated differently from those without SA. For example, it has been reported that borderline patients with SA experience difficulties when applying for treatment. Anecdotal data indicate that this group may be caught in a therapeutic "Catch-22" situation in which they cannot enter the mental health service system until they stop using substances and cannot enter substance abuse treatment until their suicidal and self-damaging behaviors are under control [14, 20, 21]. Several factors may account for this phenomenon, including: 1) segregations in the mental health field, 2) the assumption that addictive behaviors should be applied as an exclusion criterion for treatment programs and studies, and 3) program differentiation.

---

* This work was supported by the Province of Noord-Holland and ZAO Health Insurance Company in Amsterdam. We gratefully acknowledge the assistance of Eveline Rietdijk and Wijnand van der Vlist with the collection of the data.

- First, mental health centres and addiction treatment programs in some countries exist separately. This health care segregation has a strong tradition in the Netherlands where the financial support systems for mental health and substance abuse are completely separate. Unfortunately, this situation often prevents clinicians from undertaking integrated and collaborative treatments for dual diagnosis patients. Only recently we have observed some initiatives in this direction often within the framework of research projects.
- Second, scientific studies and clinical treatment programs often view addictive behaviors as an exclusion criterion for treatment of borderline personality disorder. For example, substance abusers tend to be excluded from studies examining efficacy of treatments designed to target borderline symptoms: 4 of 5 randomized controlled trials of psychosocial interventions for BPD excluded borderline patients with SA [15, 22-27]. The practise of excluding borderline patients with substance abuse is questionable given recent findings pertaining to the lack of clinical relevance of addictive behaviors among borderline patients. For example, one study recently showed that the clinical and aetiological differences between borderline patients with and without substance abuse are limited in number and size [28].
- Third, rather than eliminating substance abuse as an exclusion criteria for treatment programs, the mental health field shows a tendency toward differentiation between symptom – and disorder-specific modules. One example is DBT program designed to reduce substance abuse problems in substance-abusing borderline patients (DBT-S [29]). This type of differentiation might be indicated if implementation of regular DBT in a population of borderline patients with and without SA severely reduced the effectiveness of DBT within either one or both subgroups – e.g., through interference with the group dynamic process – or, alternatively, if treatment outcome data indicated that substance abuse is a strong predictor of poor treatment outcome for standard DBT. The most obvious disadvantage of treatment differentiation at a symptom-specific level is the enormous organisational challenge resulting from the need for a very large number of treatment modules to account for the whole clinical population.

Above we have described some of the issues that might account for the observation that borderline patients with SA experience difficulties when applying for treatment. In 1995, the Jellinek Center for substance abuse treatment and the Amsterdam Institute for Addiction Research (AIAR) started a randomized clinical trial of DBT in a mixed population of borderline patients with and without comorbid SA. Previous studies have shown that standard DBT compared to treatment-as-usual (TAU) is effective in reducing severe borderline symptomatology in borderline patients without SA [23], and that a modified version of this program (DBT-S) is effective in reducing substance abuse in borderline patients with SA [29]. Against the background of these findings, we initiated a study to evaluate whether standard DBT would also be applicable and effective in the treatment of BPD pathology and substance abuse problems.

This paper aims to examine the following research questions:

- Can standard DBT be implemented among a mixed group of borderline patients with and without SA? What specific problems are encountered and what solutions to these problems can be found?
- Is standard DBT equally efficacious in reducing borderline symptomatology among those with and those without comorbid substance abuse?
- Is standard DBT efficacious in terms of reducing the severity of the substance use problems?

Method

Aspects of implementation

A standard DBT program, focusing on life-threatening and suicidal behavior as primary treatment targets, was implemented in the Jellinek Addiction Treatment Center in Amsterdam. Female patients with borderline personality disorder were recruited from both substance abuse treatment centres and psychiatric services in the greater Amsterdam area, irrespective of the severity of their substance use problems. During a pilot phase, interviews at the beginning and the end of treatment with both patients and therapists were held to obtain information about implementation issues.

Dialectical Behavior Therapy (DBT) is a manualized 12-month treatment that combines 4 modules: 1. weekly individual cognitive-behavioral psychotherapy sessions with the primary therapist, 2. weekly skills training groups lasting 2-2.5 hours per session, 3. weekly supervision and consultation meetings for the therapists, and 4. phone consultation, where patients are encouraged to get coaching in the appliance of new effective skills by phoning their primary therapists either during or outside office hours. Individual therapy focuses primarily on motivational issues, including the motivation to stay alive and to stay in treatment. Group therapy teaches self-regulation and change skills, and self and other acceptance skills. Among its central principles is DBT's simultaneous focus on applying both acceptance and validation strategies and change (behavioural) strategies to achieve a synthetic (dialectical) balance in client functioning.

Therapists: recruitment and training

A core group of three therapists was sent to Seattle to be trained in DBT. Back in Amsterdam, they recruited additional therapists from psychiatric hospitals in Amsterdam and the Jellinek Addiction Treatment Center through introductory lectures over a two month period [30]. Therapists were invited to refer their patients, but also to take part in the project themselves as therapists. The core group therapists provided training through in-service meetings and workshops. Ongoing supervision and theoretical training were provided by the project manager (LMCvdB) in the consultation team.

Recruitment of patients

The patient group in the pilot phase consisted of nine substance-abusing (para)suicidal, and self-mutilating female borderline patients. Exclusion criteria were the identical to those used in standard DBT programs except that substance abuse was not an exclusion criterion. The average age of subjects in the pilot group was 37.5 years. The average number of days in residential treatment in the last four years was 74 days per year. The average number of admissions in the last four years ranged from 4 to 58.

Efficacy of standard DBT in a mixed group of borderline patients with or without substance abuse problems: effects on BPD symptomatology

We conducted a randomized clinical trial, comparing the efficacy of DBT with TAU in 58 female patients with borderline personality disorder. Participants were clinical referrals from both substance use treatment and psychiatric services. The inclusion criteria were: 1) DSM-IV diagnosis of BPD; 2) currently in outpatient psychiatric or substance abuse treatment; 3) age between 18 and 70; and 4) residence within a 25-mile circle around Amsterdam. Exclusion criteria were: 1) a DSM-IV diagnosis of bipolar disorder or (chronic) psychotic disorder; 2) insufficient command of the Dutch language; and 3) severe cognitive impairments. Referred patients were requested to fill out a screening device (PDQ-4+ [31]). Subsequently, patients were diagnosed using a semi-structured interview (SCID-II [32]). Substance abuse problems were assessed with the European version of the Addiction Severity Index (EuropASI [33]). Substance abuse of the participants are presented in *table I*. Patients with a severity score of 5 of higher on either the alcohol or drug section were considered substance abusers (SA+) and those with severity scores of 4 or lower on both sections were considered non-substance abusers (SA-) (*table I*).

The sample selection strategy, instrumentation, treatment conditions, and data analytic strategy and first results has been described in detail elsewhere [34]. In summary, intention-to-treat (ITT) analyses are available for 27 subjects assigned to DBT and 31 participants assigned to TAU. Outcome measures include (1) treatment retention and (2) high-risk suicidal, self-mutilative, and otherwise self-damaging impulsive behaviors. The 12-month efficacy data with respect to treatment retention and severe borderline symptomatology are reported elsewhere [34], and will be summarized below. Special attention will be paid to the long-term effects of DBT on BPD

Table I. Variation in Substance Abuse behavior among the participants.

EuropASI N = 58 Severity ratings	BPD SA +		BPD SA −	
	%	N	%	N
Cut-off score ASI ≥ 4	69%	40	31%	18
Cut-off score ASI ≥ 5	53%	31	47%	27
Cut-off score ASI ≥ 6	16%	9	84%	49

EuropASI N = 58 Severity ratings ASI ≥ 5	BPD SA +	N = 31
	%	N
Cannabis	30	9
Heroin	9	3
Cocaine	17	5
Methadone	13	4
Alcohol	50	15
Medication (sedatives)	64	19
Poly drug abuse	56	17
Average number of years of SA	7.6	
Average number of treatments	4	

symptomatology, and on the potential modification of the treatment effect of DBT on BPD symptoms by the presence of comorbid SA problems.

Efficacy of standard DBT in a mixed group of borderline patients with or without substance abuse problems: effect on SA

The efficacy of DBT in terms of the course of substance use behaviors and borderline symptomatology at 18-month follow-up will be presented.

■ Statistical Analysis

The impact of substance abuse problems on the 12-month efficacy data is analyzed using a general linear mixed model (GLMM) approach (procedure Mixed from SAS version 6.12; SAS institute, Inc, Cary, NC). To test the hypothesis (i.e., substance use modifies impact of DBT on borderline symptomatology), we used models with time, treatment, substance abuse problems, and the two-way and three-way interactions between these variables. In these analyses we focused on the treatment-by-substance abuse and time-by-treatment-by- substance abuse interactions (to inspect whether any of these were statistically significant) as well as on the treatment factor and time-by-treatment interaction (to inspect whether these were similar to the effects as observed in the models without the addiction factor).

The effect of DBT on the course of substance abuse at 18-month follow-up is examined using an analysis of variance (ANOVA) approach (SPSS version 8.0; General Linear Model Module). To test the hypothesis that DBT results in greater reductions of substance abuse problems than TAU, we used models with substance abuse severity as dependent variable, treatment as an independent variable, and initial substance abuse severity as a co-variate. In these analyses we focused of course on the treatment factor.

Results

Aspects of implementation

Experiences of patients
From the beginning, both therapists and patients expected that it would be difficult to combine substance abusing and non-substance abusing patients. Some even thought that the two groups would not mix at all over time. In reality, the two subgroups appeared to get along easily with each other by the second week. Through the discussion of homework, the substance abusing and non-substance abusing participants realized that they shared most of the essential borderline problems. Exit interviews showed that all patients judged the program as validating and helpful. They felt acknowledged as borderline patients, and judged the treatment as very important. Session attendance for the total group was 81%. No difference in attendance was found for patients with and without substance abuse problems.

Experiences of therapists in individual therapies or sessions
In the beginning, therapists seemed to belong to different worlds. Therapists recruited from the addiction field experienced difficulty staying focused on the hierarchy of borderline pathology targets. They tended to immediately turn their attention to the substance abuse as soon as it showed up in sessions, even when suicidal and self-destructive behaviors were present. Therapists recruited from the psychiatric field, however, had essentially no experience with the treatment of substance abusers other than to refer them elsewhere. Initially these therapists did not consider (severe) alcohol and medication abuse – which often lowers the threshold for (para) suicidal and self-mutilative behavior – as examples of addiction, as is drug abuse. This realization was a shock to some of them. The gaps between the two groups of therapists were closed in the consultation team meetings. At these meetings, which were focused in part on providing support to therapists through behavioural analysis, the individual therapists became aware of the many advantages of working with colleagues with different types of expertise. In addition, the combination of individual psychotherapy and group training was experienced as helpful. Phone consultation to the patient – an essential ingredient of DBT – turned out to be a serious problem, because therapists were unwilling to try this mode of treatment. Therapists were convinced that the patients would abuse the possibility of calling 24 hours a day, especially at night, and this would result in therapist burnout. Fortunately, the patients opposed this reluctance and demanded phone consultation because it was in the protocol. The concept of the patient being her own case-manager proved to be of help here. Patients were encouraged to convince their individual therapists to give phone consultation a try and this approach turned out to be successful.

Another problem resulted from the DBT rule that patients cannot be expelled from the program. In particular, the experience of patients who relapsed to substance abuse and were not referred out of the program resulted in heated discussions in the consultation team. In the end, substance abuse was redefined as a problem behavior that needs to be addressed in individual therapy sessions in order to prevent the patient from dropping out of the program. Over time, therapists in individual therapies or sessions reported feeling less isolated and more competent and also reported increased work satisfaction. The attendance rate for the consultation team was 100%.

Experiences of the group skills trainers
All the problems in the skills group were related to an initial lack of clear rules, *e.g.* with respect to substance abuse before or during the training meetings. The DBT framework does not actually provide explicit instructions to trainers on the question of whether a patient who had used substance prior to a meeting should be sent home; instead, DBT encourages trainers to rely on their own judgement. Some trainers as well as some patients expressed concern about the lack of standardized, procedures in this regard. In practise, however, there were hardly any problems with

this issue. In fact, a patient came to a session under the influence of alcohol only once during the 20 pilot training sessions. The trainers decided to let her stay because she could sit upright and utter understandable syllables and she stayed the entire session. Two weeks later, this patient reported to the trainers that she had visited her general practitioner to obtain antialcohol medication. She reported that the experience of sitting drunk in the skills group for the whole session and not being sent away had been a horrible experience. The fact that dealing directly with this patient had prevented her from dropping out made the trainers see how ineffective traditional procedures can be.

Another problem that turned up was related to the fact that all patients had been members of dynamic and interaction oriented groups. DBT involves concentrating on practising skills, rather than taking care of or discussing other patients' problems. This guideline required constant attention from the group skill trainers and a shift in attitud for most patients. For some of them, this shift was difficult to learn and at times challenging and upsetting as it made them conscious of their own judgemental behavior.

This study which is the first clinical trial that was not conducted by the developer of DBT and was conducted outside the US supports the accumulating evidence that DBT can be successfully disseminated in other settings and other countries and that mental health professionals outside academic research centres can effectively learn and apply DBT.

Efficacy of standard DBT in a mixed group of borderline patients with or without substance abuse problems: effects on BPD symptomatology

The efficacy study which will be reported extensively elsewhere [34], yielded three major results. First, DBT effectively retained patients in therapy. The 12-month attrition rate was 37% in the DBT group compared to 77% in the control condition. Second, DBT resulted in greater reductions of self-mutilating behavior and self-damaging impulsive acts than TAU. Third, the beneficial impact on the frequency of self-mutilating behaviors was far more pronounced among those who reported higher baseline frequencies of these behaviors compared with those reporting lower baseline frequencies. These results are highly concordant with previously published trials [23]. It is also important to note that this study allowed for more rigorous statistical testing of DBT's efficacy than former trials due to a relatively large sample size (N = 58).

The currently described RCT is the first study that examined the influence of comorbid SA on the efficacy of standard DBT on borderline symptomatology. The hypothesis that comorbid substance abuse modifies the impact of DBT on borderline symptomatology was rejected by the additional statistical analyses. The treatment-by-substance abuse and time-by-treatment-by-substance abuse interactions appeared to be non-significant, and adding substance use in the statistical model did not significantly alter the treatment and time-by-treatment interaction parameters. Thus, the observed favorable impact of DBT on borderline symptomatology occurred among non-substance using as well as substance using borderline patients.

Efficacy of standard DBT in a mixed group of borderline patients with or without substance abuse problems: effect on SA

Table II shows the impact of DBT, as compared to TAU, on measures of substance abuse at 18-month follow-up, corrected for initial substance use severity scores. The results indicate that no differential treatment effects were found. This is true for the number of days of alcohol, medication, and cannabis use in the past month as well as for the overall severity scores for both alcohol and drug problems. Based on these findings, the second hypothesis (*i.e.*, DBT results in greater reductions of substance use problems than TAU) should be rejected. Inspection of the findings reveals that in both treatment conditions, the course of the substance use problems is rather stable with almost no change over the 18-month follow-up period. This implies that the substance use problems were not effectively targeted in the TAU nor in the DBT condition (table II).

Table II. Impact of Dialectical Behavior Therapy on severity of substance use problems at 18-month follow-up.

Treatment condition:	Dialectical Behavior Therapy		Treatment-As-Usual		Comparison at 18-month fu corrected for baseline[2]	
EuropASI item[1]	M ± SD		M ± SD			
	Baseline n = 27	fu[3] n = 20	Baseline n = 31	fu[3] n = 24	F	p
days ≥ 5 drinks past month 0-30	7.1 ± 10.3	6.1 ± 9.8	6.2 ± 9.2	3.8 ± 7.8	0.9	.34
days medication use past month 0-30	14.2 ± 14.0	7.9 ± 12.2	13.5 + 14.5	11.5 + 13.9	0.4	.54
days cannabis use past month 0-30	6.5 ± 11.2	9.2 ± 13.3	2.3 ± 5.8	5.9 ± 11.5	0.1	.73
days alcohol problems past month 0-30	8.7 ± 12.3	7.0 ± 11.3	9.0 ± 12.9	6.7 ± 11.3	0.0	.89
days drug problems past month 0-30	8.1 ± 11.4	9.5 ± 13.2	9.0 ± 12.6	4.5 ± 10.0	2.0	.17
severity alcohol problems 0-9	2.7 ± 2.3	2.8 ± 2.6	3.0 + 2.5	2.4 ± 2.1	1.1	.31
severity drug problems 0-9	3.3 ± 2.0	2.8 ± 2.2	3.6 ± 2.3	2.3 ± 1.8	0.5	.47

1. European version of Addiction Severity Index (Kokkevi & Hartgers, 1995).
2. Using General Linear Model module of Statistical Package for Social Sciences (SPSS 8.0), with EuropASI scores at 18-month follow-up as dependent variables, treatment condition as fixed factor, and baseline scores on EuropASI as covariaties.
3. Follow-up scores at 18-months since start of treatment.

■ Discussion

This study is aimed at examining whether standard DBT can be applied to a dual diagnosis population, *i.e.* whether standard DBT can be implemented in regular mental health or regular substance abuse treatment settings for borderline patients with and without substance abuse problems. Our results indicate *(1)* the implementation process occurred without major problems, *(2)* standard DBT is as effective for substance abusing borderline patients as for non-substance abusing borderline patients when suicidal and self-destructive behavior are focus of treatment, and *(3)* standard DBT does not seem to affect the substance abuse problems in these patients.

Linehan et al. [29] developed a modified, intensified and extended version of DBT, including all the standard components, targeting substance abuse. Specific training of DBT therapists in the additional substance abuse module was a prerequisite. Koerner & Linehan [35] found DBT-S had significantly lower drop-out rates and showed significantly more reductions in drug abuse throughout the treatment year and at follow-up (16 months) compared to subjects in TAU. No differences, however, were reported for the medical or psychiatric inpatient treatment received by DBT-S and TAU subjects, nor for rates of parasuicidal behavior. Examination of the DBT-S treatment program shows that is was primarily focusing on the substance abuse rather than on high-risk suicidal and self-damaging behaviors. The focus on one target group of behavior seems to be a common trait of the other DBT programs aimed at other severe dysfunctional behaviors, such as binge eating [36, 37].

In the DBT trials published thus far, we recognize an interesting pattern: DBT is effective in terms of the specific *behavioural* target that is focused on, but this impact does not seem to generalize to behavioural domains that have not been targeted. In this sense, DBT is an example of an excellent behavior therapy program that can be effective for the treatment of severe symptomatology of serious personality pathology. This conclusion has a number of implications.

First, there is now substantial evidence that DBT is an excellent choice for patients with severe, life- or health-threatening impulse control disorders (e.g., high-risk suicidal, self-damaging, and otherwise self-damaging behaviors) that have proven to be relatively resistant to change in standard or short-term treatments. There is no empirical support that the core pathology of many patients with borderline personality disorder (i.e. chronic emptiness and boredom, unstable relationships associated with primitive defences, identity disorder, etc.) is affected by DBT (applied during one year). Perhaps, these intrapsychic elements of the pathology might benefit more from insight or psychodynamically oriented psychotherapeutic approaches (e.g.) [27, 37].

The second implication is that standard DBT can be modified such that multiple targets can be focused on, depending on the specific behavioural problems of individual patients. Our experiences in Amsterdam made clear to us that in our standard DBT program, a focus was missing: substance abuse. Therefore, we would strongly recommend integrating these potential modifications within standard DBT, rather than developing different treatment programs for distinct patients group. In particular, we would recommend that the hierarchy used in the treatment program be modified. Substance abuse should be prioritized next to or just below suicidal and self-damaging behaviors. In addition, the education of DBT therapists should include training in counselling techniques for substance abusers and strategies for modifying addictive behaviors. There are two good reasons for this recommendation:

- patients with impulse control disorders tend to have multiple problems simultaneously or, alternatively, tend to shift from one to another type of problem behavior;
- the development of symptom-specific programs would introduce an undesirably high degree of differentiation that poses an enormous, if not impossible, organisational challenge for the mental health field.

This study has a number of limitations. The sample size is rather small for studying three-way interactions; thus the analyses with respect to the possible differential impact of substance use severity on DBT's efficacy should be regarded with some caution. Furthermore, the recommendation mentioned above, i.e. to develop multi-target DBT, is basically derived from indirect evidence. Future randomized trials are required to test the relative efficacy of that approach.

In conclusion, the current study provides evidence that standard DBT can be implemented and is efficacious among both non-substance abusing and substance abusing borderline patients, but does not seem to affect substance abuse behaviors. We have recommended developing a multi-targeted DBT program for a broad patient population including several specific impulse control disorders and combinations of these disorders.

References

1. Trull TJ, Sher KJ, Minks-Brown C, Durbin J, Burr R. Borderline personality disorder and substance use disorders: A review and integration. *Clin Psych Review* 2000; 20 (2): 235-53.
2. Links PS, Heslegrave RJ, Mitton JE, van Reekum R, Patric J. Borderline psychopathology and recurrences of clinical disorders. *J Nerv Ment Dis* 1995; 183 (9): 582-6.
3. Oldham JM, Skodol AE, Kellman HD, Hyler SE, Doidge N, Rosnick L, Gallaher PE. Co-morbidity of axis I and axis II disorders. *Am J Psychiatry* 1995: 152 (4): 571-8.
4. Dulit RA, Fyer MR, Haas GL, Sullivan T, Frances AJ. Substance use in borderline personality disorder. *Am J Psychiatry* 1990; 147 (8): 1002-7.
5. Zanarini MC, Frankenburg FR, Dubo ED, Sickel AE, Trikha A, Levin A, Reynolds V. Axis I co-morbidity of borderline personality disorder. *Am J Psychiatry* 1998; 155 (12): 1733-9.
6. Zimmerman M, Coryell W. DSM-III personality disorder diagnoses in a non-patient sample. *Arch Gen Psychiatry* 1989; 46: 682-9.
7. Akiskal HS, Chen SE, Davis GC. Borderline: an adjective in search of a noun. *J Clin Psychiatry* 1985; 46: 41-8.
8. Loranger AW, & Tulis EH, Family history of alcoholism in borderline personality disorder. *Arch Gen Psychiatry* 1985; 42: 153-7.

9. Zanarini MC, Gunderson JG, Frankenburg FR, Chauncey DL. The revised diagnostic interview for borderlines: Discriminating borderline personality disorder from other axis II disorders. *J Pers Disord* 1989; 3 (1): 10-8.
10. Zanarini MC, Gunderson JG, Frankenburg FR, Chauncey DL. Discriminating borderline personality disorder from other axis II disorders. *Am J Psychiatry* 1990; 147: 161-7.
11. Zanarini MC. Borderline personality disorder as an impulse spectrum disorder. In: Paris P, ed. *Borderline personality disorder: aetiology and treatment*. Washington, DC: American Psychiatric Press, 1993: 67-86.
12. Verheul R, van den Brink W, Hartgers C. Prevalence of personality disorders among alcoholics and drug addicts: an overview. *Eur Addict Res* 1995; 1: 166-77.
13. Rounsaville BJ, Kranzler HR, Ball S, Tennen H, Poling J, Triffleman E. Personality disorders in substance abusers: Relation to substance use. *J Nerv Ment Dis* 1998; 186 (2): 87-95.
14. Verheul R, Ball S, Brink W van den. Substance abuse and personality disorders. In: Kranzler HR, Rounsaville BJ, eds. *Dual diagnosis and treatment: substance abuse and comorbid medical and psychiatric disorders*. New York, NY: Marcel Dekker, Inc., 1997: 317-63.
15. Linehan MM, Armstrong HE, Suarez A, Allmon D, Heard, HL. Cognitive-behavioural treatment of chronically parasuicidal borderline patients. *Arch Gen Psychiatry* 1991; 48: 1060-4.
16. Linehan MM, Heard HL, Armstrong HE. Naturalistic follow-up of a behavioural treatment for chronically parasuicidal borderline patients. *Arch Gen Psychiatry* 1993; 50: 971-4.
17. Siever LJ, Davis KL. A psychobiological perspective on the personality disorders. *Am J Psychiatry* 1991; 148: 1647-58.
18. Reekum R van, Links PS, Fedorov C. Impulsivity in borderline personality disorder. In: Silk KR, ed. *Biological and neurobehavioural studies of borderline personality disorder*. Washington, DC: American Psychiatric Press, 1994: 1-22.
19. Links PS, Heslegrave R, van Reekum R. Impulsivity: core aspect of borderline personality disorder. *J Pers Disord* 1999; 13: 1-9.
20. Bosch LMC van den. Dialectische gedragstherapie bij verslaafden met een BPS. In: *Handboek Verslaving* (B 4375-1). Houten: Bohn Stafleu Van Loghum, 1996.
21. NIAAA (National Institute of Alcohol Abuse and Alcoholism). Psychiatric co-morbidity with alcohol use disorders. In: *Eighth special report to the US congress on alcohol and health*. NIAAA, 1993: 37-59.
22. Evans K, Tyrer P, Catalan J, Schmidt U, Davidson K, Dent J, Tata P, Thornton S, Barber J, Thompson S. Manual-assisted cognitive-behaviour therapy (MACT): A randomised controlled trial of a brief intervention with bibliotherapy in the treatment of recurrent deliberate self-harm. *Psychol Med* 1999; 29: 19-25.
23. Linehan MM. *Cognitive behavioural treatment of borderline personality disorder*. New York, NY: Guilford Press, 1993b.
24. Linehan MM, Dimeff LA. *Dialectical Behaviour Therapy Manual of Treatment Interventions for Drus Abusers with Borderline Personality Disorder*. Seattle, Washington: University of Washington, 1997.
25. Linehan MM, Comtois KA, Koerner K, et al. University of Washington study of Dialectical Behaviour Therapy: a preliminary report. Paper presented at the meeting of the Association of Advancement of Behaviour Therapy. Washington, DC: 1998.
26. Marziali E, Munroe-Blum H. *Interpersonal Group Psychotherapy for Borderline Personality Disorder*. New York: Basic Books, 1994.
27. Bateman A, Fonagy P. The effectiveness of partial hospitalization in the treatment of Borderline Personality Disorder: a randomised controlled trial. *Am J Psychiatry* 1999; 156: 1563-9.
28. Bosch LMC van den, Verheul R, Brink W van den. Substance Abuse in Borderline Personality Disorder: Clinical and Etiological Correlates. *J Pers Disord* 2001; 15 (5): 416-24.
29. Linehan MM, Schmidt H, Dimeff LA, Craft JC, Kanter J, Comtois KA. Dialectical behaviour therapy for patients with borderline personality disorder and drug-dependence. *Am J Addiction* 1999; 8 (4): 279-92.
30. Bosch W van den, Egberts T, Ingenhoven Th, Kuipers H. Tussen Amsterdam en Seattle: de methode Linehan. In: *MGV* 1995; 50 (10): 1096-103.

31. Hyler SE. *Personality Diagnostic Questionnaire, DSM-IV version (PDQ-4+)* [Dutch translation by Akkerhuis GW, et al., 1996]. New York, NY: New York State Psychiatric Institute, 1994.
32. First MB, Spitzer RL, Gibbon M, et al. *Structured Clinical Interview for DSM-IV Axis II Personality Disorders (SCID-II, Version 2.0)* [Dutch translation by Weertman A, et al., 1996]. New York, NY: Biometrics Research Department, New York State Psychiatric Institute, 1994.
33. Kokkevi A, Hartgers C. EuropASI: European adaptation of a multidimensional assessment instrument for drug and alcohol dependence. *Eur Addict Res* 1995; 1: 208-10.
34. Verheul R, Bosch LMC van den, Koeter MWJ, Ridder MAJ de, Stijnen T, Brink W van den. A 12-month randomized clinical trial of Dialectical Behaviour Therapy for women with borderline personality disorder in the Netherlands. (submitted).
35. Koerner K, Dimeff LA. Further data on Dialectical Behaviour Therapy. *Clinical Psychology: science and practise.* 2000; Spring: 104-12.
36. Koerner K, Linehan MM. Research on Dialectical Behaviour Therapy for patients with borderline personality disorder. *Psychiatr Clin North Am* 2000; 23: 151-67.
37. Young JE. *Cognitive therapy for personality disorders: A schema-focused approach.* Revised edition. Sarasota: Professional Resource Press; 1994.

The integral care programme for sick physicians (PAIMM) of the medical council of Barcelona

P. Lusilla[2], E. Bruguera[1,2], A. Arteman[2], A. Gual[1,3], M. Martínez[2], V. Marcos[2], G. Escuder[1,2], J. Matalí[1,2], C. Roncero[1,2], A. Ramos[1,2], F. Collazos[1,2], P. Duro[2], A. Blasi[1,2], J. Padrós[2], M. Casas[1,2]

1. Department of Psychiatry. University General Hospital Vall d'Hebrón of Barcelona
2. PAIMM, Medical Council of Barcelona
3. Alcohol Unit, Hospital Clínic of Barcelona

■ Definition

The PAIMM is a programme devoted to assisting physicians who suffer from mental disorders and/or who are addicted to alcohol and/or other substances, including psychopharmaceutical products. The rationale for the programme is based on the observation that impaired doctors tend to hide such problems on the one hand and refrain from seeking medical help on the other, the combination of which can easily result in their providing less than adequate medical care, thereby jeopardizing the health of their patients.

The programme was jointly created in 1998 by the Department of Health of the Regional Government of Catalonia and the Catalan Medical Association, and is managed by the Medical Council of Barcelona. The Psychiatric Services Department of Vall d'Hebron University Hospital also provides support to the programme.

Table I shows the important events related to the PAIMM.

Table I. Important events in PAIMM.

- November 1998: Initiation of ambulatory consultations
- March 1999: Inpatient unit (8 beds) established
- April 2000: Agreement with the main health
- care service providers signed
- September 2000: Creation of RETURN, by The Catalonia Nurses Association
- June 2001: Day hospital established
- August 2001: Growth of inpatient Unit to 13 beds

Background

Programmes for impaired physicians began in United States and Canada in the eighties as it had been discovered that health professionals in general, and doctors in particular, often fail to take the necessary steps to ensure their health [1, 2]. It is important to keep in mind that mental and addictive illnesses still have a strong social stigma attached to them, even within the health community. Within the medical field, some hold the view that suffering from an illness is an indication of weakness. For doctors who suffer from such problems, fear of detection by co-workers or by patients plays an important dissuasive role against seeking help. In such cases, there is a strong tendency to experience these illnesses with feelings of guilt, and an equally strong tendency to hide the illnesses, which combine to delay seeking help and to worsen the prognosis.

Table II. Specialties for Inpatients Doctors.

Medical Specialties Doctors	
General Practitioner	41%
Psychiatry	11%
Pediatry	5%
Resident	5%
Internal Medicine	5%
Intensive Medicine	3%
Odontology	3%
Microbiology	2%
Anesthesiology	2%
Haematology	2%
Occupational medicine	2%
Recently Graduated	2%
Other specialties	13%

Purposes of PAIMM

The aim of the programme is to rehabilitate doctors and facilitate their return to work. It is in accordance with the Code of Conduct (Norms of Medical Ethics) to improve the quality of medical care received by the public on the one hand, and on the other to help physicians achieve an optimal professional practise.

Are these kinds of programme really useful?

The utility of programmes dedicated to the treatment of sick doctors is based on the combined problems of increased health risk and fear of seeking help. Research indicates that many doctors are not concerned about their health; 50% of those surveyed in Catalonia do not have a general practitioner [3]. Other research indicates that 70% suffer from stress symptoms, and those with substance abuse problems delay seeking help for up to six or seven years [4]. Physicians suffering from severe depression, are rarely admitted to a psychiatric unit, which is most likely related to the high suicide rate of this population [5-7]. These findings demonstrate that doctors' reticence to seek help may result serious consequences, as can be seen in *Figure 1*.

The usefulness of these programmes has also been demonstrated in the research literature, which describes high rates of recovery; rehabilitation rates amongst addicted doctors is 75-88% over five years, while that of the general population is 66% [7].

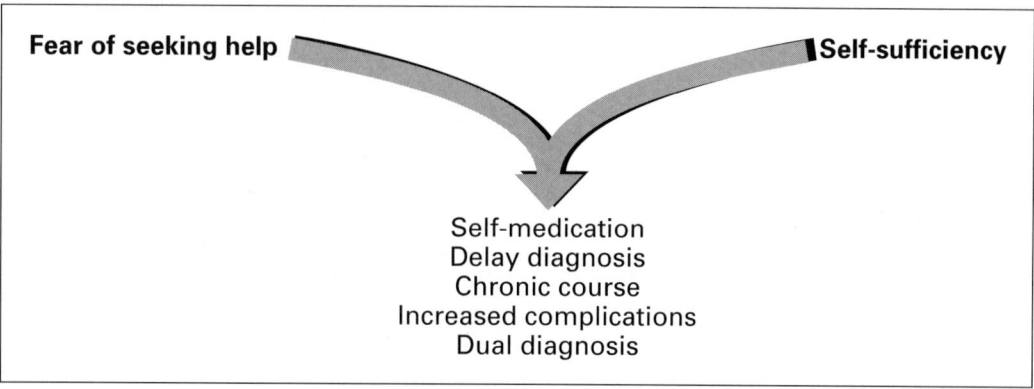

Figure 1. Risk of sick physicians.

Table III. Diagnosis (DSM IV criteria)*.

Psychiatric diagnosis	
Major depression	24.5%
Bipolar disorder	12.2%
Personality disorder	6.2%
Eating disorder	5.4%
Adaptive disorder	3.4%
Anxiety disorder	2.8%
Gambling disorder	2%
Obsessive-Compulsive dis.	1.4%
Schizoaffective disorder	1.4%
Brief Psychotic episode	1.4%
Delirant chronic disorder	1.4%
Schizophrenia	0.7%
Drug related diagnosis	
Alcohol	49%
Cocaine	9.2%
Opiates	9.5%
Benzodiazepines	9.5%
Amphetamines	1.4%
Cannabinoids	0.7%
Other psychiatric conditions	
Suicidal attempt	4.8%
Suicidal thoughts	2.7%

(*) Some patients have more than one diagnosis.

■ Characteristics of PAIMM

The main features of the programme include:
- Confidentiality, which is strictly guaranteed at all times.
- Integral services: including outpatient treatment, a day hospital and an inpatient unit.
- Family assistance.
- Social assistance.
- Legal support.
- Job-related assistance.

Services are free to physicians licensed in Catalonia and in associated Regions. Since September 2000, the programme has offered identical services to sick nurses (the RETORN programme). The philosophy of PAIMM can be outlined in the four points that follow:

- Preventive.
- Non punitive (unless necessary).
- Promoting voluntary access.
- Promoting rehabilitation and return to work.

As such, "compulsory" access to the programme (after an official complaint) is decreasing, as indicated in *Figure 2*.

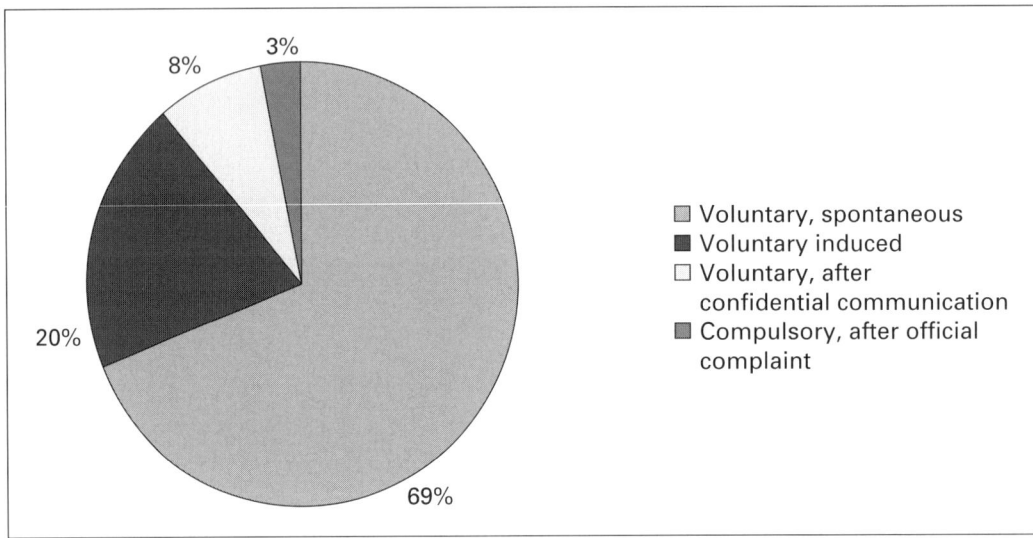

Figure 2. Mode of access to PAIMM.

Services to the sick doctor are always provided with informed consent at the outset, and treatment strategies include therapeutic contracts. The Therapeutic Contract could be type I or type II. The first is only between the patient and therapist whereas type II is between the patient and therapist as well as with the Medical Association.

■ The structure and treatment strategies of the PAIMM

Figure 3 shows the structure of PAIMM. The team is composed of ten psychiatrists and five psychologists who provide support at the different assistance levels. There are three more doctors available from Central Services, which also provides an internist and specialized nurses to the inpatient unit.

At the Clinical Units the treatment goals include:

- Detoxification and rehabilitation of addictive behaviour.
- Integral (psychological and psychopharmacological) care of mental disorders.
- Diagnostic evaluation.

The treatment strategies include: careful medical and psychological examination, prevention strategies (educational and *social life skills* to address problems), programmes to raise awareness regarding the danger of self-medication with prescription drugs, family support, group therapy, and drug screening. The therapeutic process is monitored via systematic quality control and patient feedback.

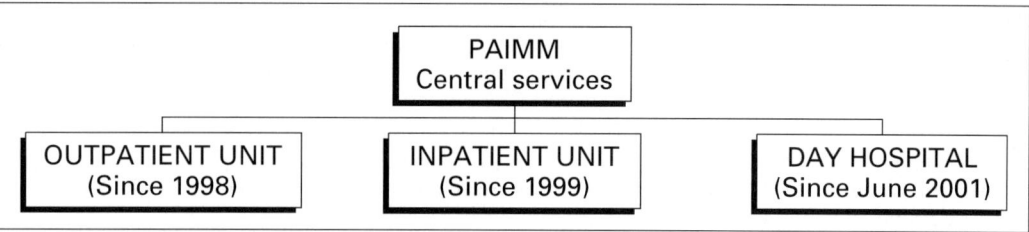

Figure 3. The structure of PAIMM.

The core of the programme is clinical care, however it includes other aspects. Central Services are very important because they provide presentations about the Programme to hospital boards, primary health care teams and other private and public organizations. Also, Central Services establish service agreements with other Autonomous Communities and Medical Councils in Spain, and with other European Countries. Finally, they direct the case management of doctors not yet admitted to the programme.

■ Clinical activity

From November 1998 to December 2002, 469 patients were admitted to the PAIMM, of which 55% were men and 45% women. The average age was as follows: 75% were between 35-55 years, and 50% were between 40-50 years of age; a large number were in their midlife work. Most of them came from Catalonia (370), 98 came from the rest of Spain and one doctor from Portugal.

Admission to the inpatient unit includes both patients from the PAIMM outpatient unit and patients from other parts of Spain. *Figure 4* shows some inpatient unit clinical activity data. Between November 1998 and December 2002, there were 294 admissions and 67 readmissions. Most of patients were men (65% male and 35% female) with an average age of 45.8 years (SD = 9.1; range = 26-72 years) and an average length of stay of 29.02 days (SD = 16.75). Total number of inpatients was 227 *(Figure 4)*.

Doctors comprised 84% of the patients, with nurses making up the remaining 16%. Amongst the doctors, the specialties mostly frequently admitted were General Practitioners (41%) and Psychiatrists (11%). *Table II* shows the specialities of the doctors admitted to the inpatient ward.

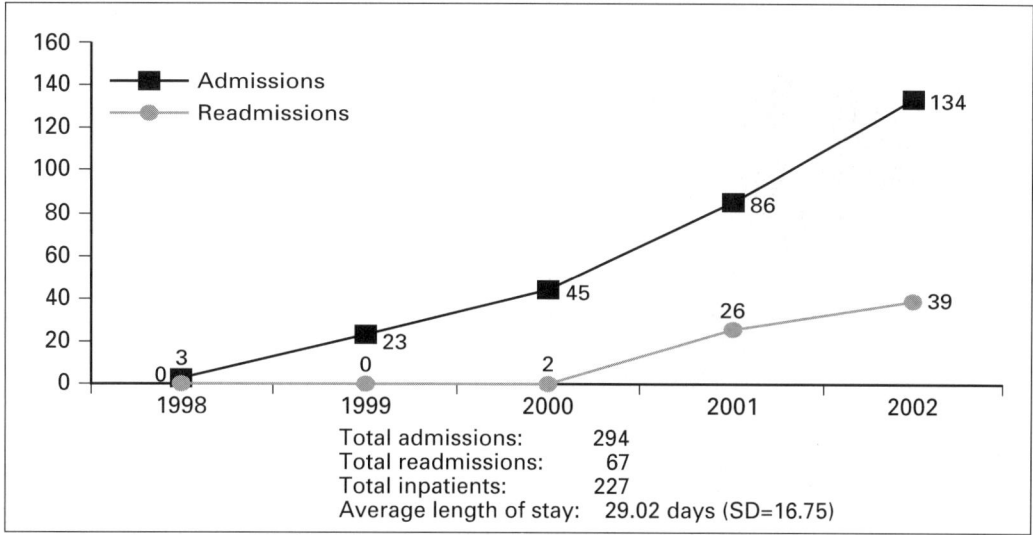

Figure 4. Descriptive analysis of admissions November 1999-December 2002.

Figure 5 shows the principal diagnosis by groups of admissions. Two thirds of the inpatients were diagnosed with substance abuse and/or dependence; 28% suffered from alcohol dependence, 16% from other drug addiction and 24% were dually diagnosed (addiction and mental disorder), with alcohol being the most commonly abused substance among the latter group. The rest of the cases (32%) were diagnosed with a mental disorder only.

Specific diagnosis by DSM IV criteria are shown in *table III*. A diagnosis of an affective disorder was the most common amongst patients suffering from a mental disorder. These results are similar to those found in other studies [8, 9].

Upon discharge from the hospital, patients completed a quality of assistance received inquiry (shown in *Figure 6*). Most indicated that they were very satisfied with the treatment in the programme.

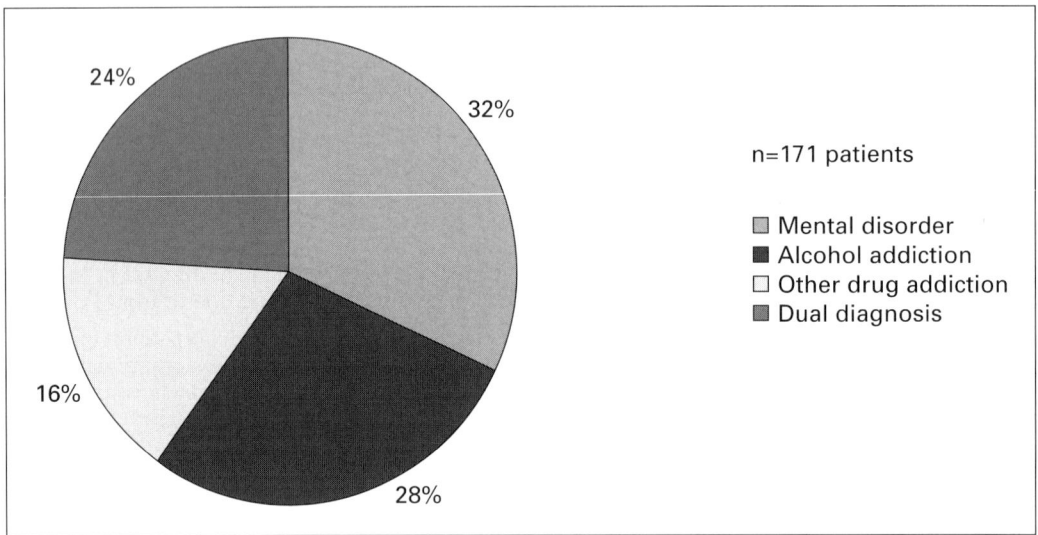

Figure 5. Admissions: Principal Diagnosis by Groups.

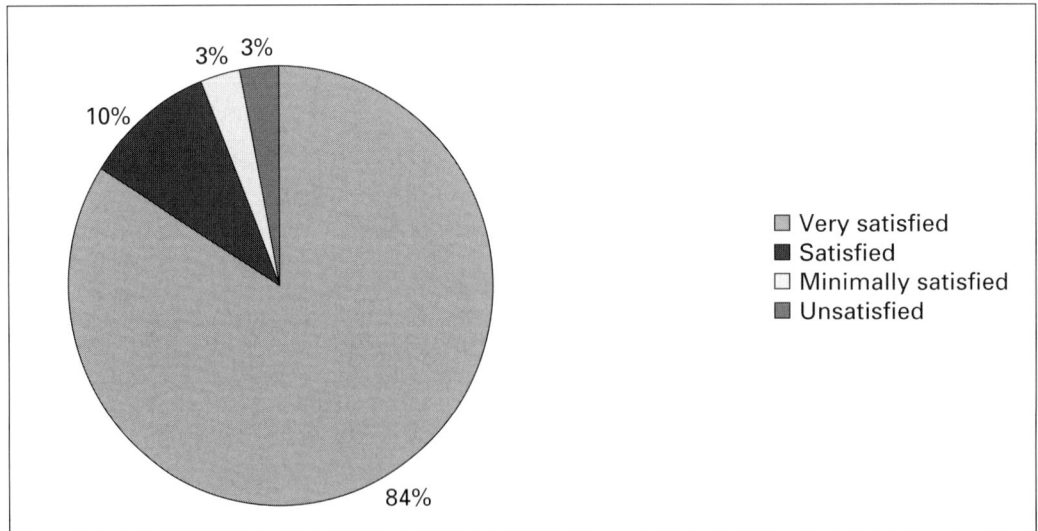

Figure 6. Satisfaction with the Program.

■ Conclusions

PAIMM is the only programme in Spain specialized to provide confidential treatment for health professionals with addiction and/or mental disorders. Since 1998 over 469 patients have received assistance. At the time of admission, most suffered from affective disorders, alcohol dependence or both. Current results are good, showing a high level of treatment compliance and very high patient satisfaction with delivery of services It should be noted that interest of this kind of programme – sick health professional – is not only an individual but also a general health issue [10].

References

1. American Medical Association. Council on mental health. The sick physicians, impairment by psychiatric disorders including alcoholism and drug dependence. JAMA 1973; 223: 684-7.
2. Talbott GD. Gallegos KV, Wilson Po, Porter TL. The medical Association of Georgia's Impaired Physicians Program. Review of the first 1,000 physicians: analysis of specialty. JAMA 1987; 257 (21): 2979-30.
3. Bruguera M, Guri J, Arteman A, Grau J, Carbonell J. *The attitude of doctors to the care of their own health.* Paper presented in the 2002 AMA/CMA International Conference on Physician Health. Vancouver, October 2002.
4. Brooke D, Edwards G, Taylor C. Addiction as an occupational hazard: 144 doctors with drug and alcohol problems. *Br J Addict* 1991; 86 (8): 1011-6.
5. Lindeman S. Suicide among physicians (dissertation) Oulu University press; 1997.
6. Lindeman S, Läärä E, Hakko H, Lönnqvist J. A systematic review on gender-specific suicide mortality in medical doctors. *Br J Psychiatry* 1996; 168: 274-9.
7. Aasland OG, Ekeberg Ø, Schweder T. Suicide rates from 1960 to 1989 in Norwegian physicians compared with other educational groups. *Social Science and Medicine* 2001; 52: 259-66.
8. Murray RM. Psychiatric illness in male doctors and controls: an analysis of Scottish hospitals inpatient data. *Br J Psychiatry* 1997; 131: 1-10.
9. Roness A, Kaldestad E. Mental disorders among physicians hospitalized in a psychiatric clinic. *Tidsskr Nor Laegeforen* 1991; 111 (30): 3619-22.
10. *Manifesto of Barcelona.* Produced by consensus in the 1st European Meeting PAIMM 2001 by expert participants about Care Programmes in Europe for health professionals with mental disorders and addictive behaviours. Barcelona, November 2001.

36-month follow up of opiate dependents in three levels of treatment intensity

M. Clerici[1], G. Carrà[2]

1. Department of Psychiatry, San Paolo's Hospital Medical School, University of Milan
2. Department of Applied Health and Behavioural Sciences, Section of Psychiatry, University of Pavia

---

Over the past two decades there has been a growing awareness of the problem of co-occurring substance use disorders in persons with severe mental illness, which is often termed dual diagnosis, because of a range adverse effects in the course of illness, service use and outcome [1].

The bulk of evidence comes from North America [2, 3] where the need for integrated mental health and substance abuse treatment services is emphasized [4]. Such programmes require additional resources and radical redesign of service delivery systems through the use of multidisciplinary teams that include both mental health and substance abuse specialists who share responsibility for treatment and a common administrative structure and funding streams. Nevertheless the current momentum for integrated programmes is not based on any clear evidence that they lead to a better outcome [5]. Furthermore in many European countries, where sector community mental health teams are well established and addiction treatment services are often inside the same administrative structure as the mental health system, the obstacles for integrated care might be fewer. A more modest and achievable strategy of diminishing fragmentation would thus be to develop closer links between addiction treatment and general adult services [6], providing special training in addiction psychiatry for some mental health staff, spending no or few extra resources for new integrated programmes.

It appears that the multi-modal biopsychosocial approach [7, 8] will be able to provide great advantages in terms of resources for the treatment of co-occurring substance abuse. These advantages range from the coordinated work of various professionals to technical and typological resources of the services, to the projection and experimentation of mainly integrated intervention models, with varying therapeutic intensities, to respond to different needs.

■ Aims

The main purpose of this study is to verify the association between treatment intensity and related retention and outcome in three different levels of treatment for opioid dependents. A secondary purpose is to examine differences in psychiatric diagnoses between patients seeking a more intensive level of treatment.

Material and methods

Study design

We carried out a clinical trial among heroin dependents with and without a co-morbidity of severe mental illness, and participating in three different levels of treatment intensity, to verify the influence of treatment intensity on treatment retention and outcome.

Setting

The study was carried out among opioid-dependent patients seeking treatment and consecutively admitted, over a period of seven years, in two NHS addicts' outpatient clinics and in a nonprofit agency for TC programs located in Milan, which directly provide and refer for further treatment for the population of Greater Milan.

The study predicted the division of the aggregate sample into three sub-groups according to their level of treatment.

Level I corresponds to patients who have received treatment in the form of:

- outpatient methadone maintenance program, paired with non-continuing monthly checkups;
- individual outpatient psycho-dynamic therapy (at least six months of continuous psychotherapy for a total of at least 20 sessions);
- outpatient group psycho-educational therapy to prepare patients for residential treatment depending on patients' motivation to enter TC program (no more than 20 sessions).

Level II focuses on subjects who have access to the following treatments:

- outpatient methadone maintenance program combined with continuous individual psychological checkups (no fewer than 20 sessions) or individual psycho-dynamic therapy treatments (no fewer than 20 sessions);
- outpatient group psycho-educational therapy to prepare patients for residential treatment depending on patients' motivation to enter TC program, also including family participation in support groups (the psychotherapy and family therapy sessions should not be fewer than 20 sessions each);
- residential drug-addiction treatment combined with thrice weekly cognitive group psychotherapy (for a duration of no longer than 6 months).

Level III focuses on patients who have received either outpatient group psycho-educational therapy for no fewer than 20 basic/introductory sessions, or 6 months of residential treatment combined with thrice weekly cognitive group psychotherapy in which time the family has taken advantage of basic/introductory support-group therapy (no fewer than 20 sessions total, five of which to be multifamily sessions).

Subjects

Overall 544 patients were admitted into three different levels of treatment. Most of them were male (76%), with a mean age of 24.4 years (s.d. = 0.6) and a lifetime substance abuse of 5.4 years (s.d. = 0.52). Most patients were single (87%). Primary education had been provided to 397 (73%) compared to 147 who obtained a high school diploma (27%).

Measures

Clinical psychiatric diagnoses, obtained at admission, were based on assessments by clinicians using DSM III-R criteria [9], and an extensive baseline interview addressed patients' demographic health and social characteristics. The patients were divided into the following 4 sub-groups according to their diagnostic profile:

- the first sub-group was composed of subjects suffering from substance abuse without an added diagnosis of mental illness (Substance Use Disorders-SU);
- the second sub-group was composed of subjects suffering from substance abuse with a diagnosis of Axis I for schizophrenia or of Axis II for cluster A personality disorders (Severe mental illness + Substance Use Disorders-SMI + SU);

- the third sub-group was composed of subjects suffering from substance abuse with a diagnosis of Axis II for cluster B and C personality disorders and a diagnosis of Axis I for mood disorders (Personality or Mood + Substance Use Disorders-PMD + SU);
- the fourth sub-group was composed of subjects suffering from substance abuse with a diagnosis of multiple psychiatric disorders (Multiple Psychiatric Disorders + Substance Use Disorders-MPD + SU).

Patients were contacted, at different times according to admission, 36 months after program completion, to be assessed for follow-up treatment. An appropriate questionnaire was administered that explored two different areas:

Retention of treatment that was defined in four major steps:

- *graduates* who completed treatment successfully according to the service staff (over 12 months of therapy);
- *self-terminators* who completed the minimum 6 months of therapy without finishing the full year as per the suggestion of the staff;
- *drop-outs* who quit the program before the minimum 6 months contrary to the suggestions of the staff. In the case of those in residential treatment, this period includes the outpatient, basic/introductory phase that precedes the residential phase;
- *extended treatment* who, at the 3-year follow-up were still in treatment with a clinic involved in the study or had switched to another clinic with the approval of their original clinic's therapy team.

Clinical outcomes, defined in three major steps:

- abstinence;
- *relapse*, i.e. constant or periodic resumption of substance use, incarceration, death, a demand for his/her re-entry into treatment;
- and *extended treatment*, which identifies those who, at the 3-year follow-up were still in treatment with one of the clinics involved in the study or had switched to another clinic with the approval of their original clinic's therapy team.

Statistical analysis

Comparisons between subgroups were performed using two-sample tests for continuous variables and chi-square tests for nominal variables, as appropriate, to analyse differences in proportions. The statistical package Stata 7.0 (Stata Corporation, 2001) was used for these analyses.

■ Results

Psychiatric diagnoses in different levels of treatment intensity

As displayed in *table I*, the global sample shows statistically significant differences in relation to treatment intensity delivered for different psychiatric subgroups ($x^2 = 12.24$, df = 6, p = 0.016). As psychiatric co-morbidity increases, the percentage of subjects who request higher level treatment intensity also increases. For example, SU patients prefer (54%) treatment intensity I compared to MPD + SU patients who are mostly (57%) engaged in treatment intensity II. From the analyses of residential and outpatient sub-groups, *table II* shows that this distribution can be attributed to the outpatient sub-group ($x^2 = 16.091$, df = 3, p = 0.001) in which SU patients prefer (71%) treatment intensity I compared to SMI + SU (65%), MPD + SU (58%) and PMD + SU (55%) who are mostly engaged in treatment intensity II.

Table I. Psychiatric diagnoses in different levels of treatment intensity (N = 544).

DSM IV diagnoses	Treatment intensity-I (N = 245) N (%)	Treatment intensity-II (N = 205) N (%)	Treatment intensity-III (N = 94) N (%)	Total	p
SU	72 (54)	38 (29)	22 (17)	132	
SMI + SU	42 (46)	34 (37)	14 (17)	90	
PMD + SU	122 (41)	118 (40)	56 (19)	296	
MPD + SU	9 (34)	15 (57)	2 (9)	26	0.016

SU = Substance Use Disorders. SMI + SU = Severe mental illness + Substance Use Disorders. PMD + SU = Personality (cluster B, C) or Mood + Substance Use Disorders. MPD + SU = Multiple Psychiatric Substance Use Disorders.

Table II. Psychiatric diagnoses in residential (N = 314) and outpatient (N = 230) subgroups in different levels of treatment intensity.

DSM IV diagnoses	Treatment intensity-I	Treatment intensity-II	Treatment intensity-III	Total	p
Residential	(N = 128) N (%)	(N = 92) N (%)	(N = 94) N (%)		
SU	21 (35)	17 (28)	22 (37)	60	
SMI + SU	32 (52)	16 (26)	14 (22)	62	
PMD + SU	72 (39)	57 (31)	56 (30)	185	
MPD + SU	3 (42)	2 (29)	2 (29)	7	NS
Outpatient	(N = 119) N (%)	(N = 111) N (%)			
SU	51 (71)	21 (29)	–	72	
SMI + SU	10 (35)	18 (65)	–	28	
PMD + SU	50 (45)	61 (55)	–	111	
MPD + SU	8 (42)	11 (58)	–	19	0.001

SU = Substance Use Disorders. SMI + SU = Severe mental illness + Substance Use Disorders. PMD + SU = Personality (cluster B, C) or Mood + Substance Use Disorders. MPD + SU = Multiple Psychiatric Substance Use Disorders.

Treatment retention and clinical outcome in different levels of treatment intensity

The follow-up was carried out on 418 subjects (rate of findings 76.7%).

However one considers the correlations among different typologies of treatment retention and levels of treatment intensity in the aggregate group ($x^2 = 210.055$, df = 4, p = 0.000), *table III*, or among the sub-groups: residential ($x^2 = 202.173$, df = 2, p = 0.000), and outpatient ($x^2 = 19.594$, df = 2, p = 0.000), *table IV*, the drop-out rates are inversely correlated to the level of treatment intensity. It is also interesting to note that 313 subjects, or 57%, have been shown to be able to take advantage of their treatment if it was of 6 months or more. Six months is the threshold for what are considered significant results of a treated group *versus* an untreated control group.

Table V Shows that clinical outcomes are significantly related ($x^2 = 50.056$, df = 4, p = 0.000) to different levels of treatment intensity in the global sample, mainly because the relapse rates are higher in less integrated treatment programs. Nevertheless it is ascribable only to the residential

Table III. Treatment retention in different levels of treatment intensity (N = 544).

Treatment retention	Treatment intensity-I (N = 253) N (%)	Treatment intensity-II (N = 198) N (%)	Treatment intensity-III (N = 93) N (%)	Total	p
Drop-out	179 (77)	47 (20)	5 (3)	231	
Graduates + self-terminators	44 (16)	133 (50)	88 (34)	265	
Extended treatment	30 (62)	18 (38)	–	48	0.000

Table IV. Treatment retention in residential (N = 314) and outpatient (N = 230) subgroups in different levels of treatment intensity.

Treatment retention	Treatment intensity-I	Treatment intensity-II	Treatment intensity-III	Total	p
Residential	(N = 130) N (%)	(N = 91) N (%)	(N = 93) N (%)		
Drop-out	122 (83)	20 (13)	5 (4)	147	
Graduates + self-terminators	8 (5)	71 (42)	88 (53)	167	
Extended treatment	–	–	–		0.000
Outpatient	(N = 123) N (%)	(N = 107) N (%)			
Drop-out	57 (67)	27 (33)	–	84	
Graduates + self-terminators	36 (37)	62 (63)	–	98	
Extended treatment	30 (62)	18 (38)	–	48	0.000

Table V. Clinical outcomes in different levels of treatment intensity (N = 418).

36 month Follow-up	Treatment intensity-I (N = 178) N (%)	Treatment intensity-II (N = 148) N (%)	Treatment intensity-III (N = 92) N (%)	Total	p
Abstinence	36 (23)	62 (40)	57 (37)	155	
Relapse	133 (54)	82 (33)	30 (13)	245	
Extended treatment	9 (50)	4 (22)	5 (28)	18	0.000

subgroup (x^2 = 49.577, df = 4, p = 0.000) as displayed in table VI, because the outpatient subgroup does not show any significant outcome difference regardless of the level of intensity and integration in treatment. Furthermore it should be emphasized that global rates of successful treatment (abstinence plus extended treatment) are around 60-70% for all treatment intensity options.

Table VI. Clinical outcome in residential (N = 314) and outpatient (N = 104) subgroups in different levels of treatment intensity.

36 month Follow-up	Treatment intensity-I	Treatment intensity-II	Treatment intensity-III	Total	p
Residential	(N = 128) N (%)	(N = 94) (%)	(N = 92) N (%)		
Abstinence	23 (83)	48 (13)	57 (4)	128	
Relapse	96 (57)	42 (25)	30 (18)	168	
Extended treatment	9 (50)	4 (22)	5 (28)	18	0.000
Outpatient	(N = 50) N (%)	(N = 54) N (%)			
Abstinence	13 (67)	14 (33)	–	27	
Relapse	37 (37)	40 (63)	–	77	
Extended treatment	–	–	–	–	NS

■ Discussion

Our study sought to examine the association between treatment intensity, related retention and outcome in three different levels of treatment for opioid dependents with and without severe mental illness. This framework implies that our results should be interpreted with caution for a number of reasons. One major limitation is that behavioural retention and outcome measures are not standardised through validated instruments nor hair and urine analyses. Moreover, the diagnoses used are clinical DSM III-R diagnoses, made by the treating psychiatrist based on signs, symptoms and history – not research diagnoses. Thus, concerns regarding the validity and reliability of the diagnoses are pertinent. Furthermore this is a service-based study, *i.e.* participants are not randomly selected but referred with potential related bias. Changes cannot necessarily be ascribed to intervention, and may reflect spontaneous improvement.

Thanks to some of the results in this study, we seem to be able to affirm that subjects with mental illness as well as substance abuse issues should have constant access to treatment. Especially in Italy today, there are early diagnosis possibilities, structured treatment and a wide variety of therapeutic resources. These resources can be directed to substitutive programs that work in conjunction with the risk reduction strategies and psycho-pharmacological medications that are useful in the treatment of psychiatric co-morbidity with substance abuse issues. The resources can also serve family therapy and psychotherapy. These treatments and the techniques suitable for them should be more integrated in the standard treatment of the patient. In this way they can facilitate the work of the service operators and can guarantee the necessary follow-up evaluations. The results we have lead us to believe, at least at first sight, that the "lowest" level of therapeutic intensity offers a lesser guarantee of effective adhesion to the program. This is generally provable today in the clinical practice of most substance abuse services that operate with a risk-reduction policy. At the same time, one should not entirely favour evaluation tendencies that rely on compliance with the treatment program. Rather, one should pay attention to the important motivational factors influencing patients and the processes of change necessary to overcome drug addiction symptoms and to reduce relapses due to psychopathological co-morbidity. In our study, the number of drop-outs seems to reduce progressively and drastically when patients take advantage of a valid and composite therapy program. This holds independent of the settings used.

If we now understand the co-morbidity phenomenon, we can also claim that the "pure" sub-group tends to take advantage of the lowest level of therapy integration in the ambulatory services. The trend for the co-morbidity sub-groups (at least among those presented here) is toward a composite treatment.

The results of the most important international follow-up research applied to substance dependency treatment [10] underline how the predictive variable of "success" is the ability to stay in treatment. If we start from the supposition that "the more a patient stays in treatment, the greater his/her chances for therapeutic success at the follow-up", it becomes clear that therapeutic integration can aid motivational reinforcement for compliance with the therapy program and can help sustain the process of change. In both cases, a result seems to have been reached: the patients' ability to prolong the therapy program and to significantly improve their adhesion to the programs, or to use sustaining techniques, are key factors in the recovery success rate.

We are therefore not yet able to "measure" if therapeutic integration of diverse psychotherapy and family therapy techniques is effective on its own or only in that it increases the length of the therapy program. The current work model, which is mainly sequential, but hopefully will soon be truly integrated on the base of specific criteria, can be amply discussed in its projection and constantly adapted over time. The specific techniques that constitute and shape the work model should certainly be refined in function of their greater compatibility, especially in regards to the psychotherapy and family therapy components. The tendency, however, increasingly points to a recognition of the clinical advantages of the integrated multi-modal bio psychosocial approach for substance abuse-related conditions [11]. A tendency that this preliminary study supports and strengthens.

References

1. Drake RE, McLaughlin P, Pepper B, Minkoff K. Dual diagnosis of major mental illness and substance disorder: an overview. In: Minkoff K, Drake RE, eds. *New Directions for Mental Health Services 50: Dual Diagnosis of Major Mental Illness and Substance Disorder.* New York: John Wiley & Sons, 1991.
2. Drake RE, Mercer-McFadden C, Mueser KT, McHugo GJ, Bond G. Review of integrated mental health and substance abuse treatment for patients with dual disorders. *Schizophr Bull* 1998; 24(4): 589-608.
3. Drake RE, Mueser KT. Psychosocial approaches to dual diagnosis. *Schizophr Bull* 2000; 26 (1): 105-18.
4. Mercer CC, Mueser KT, Drake RE. Organizational guidelines for dual disorders programs. *Psychiatric Quarterly* 1998; 69: 145-68.
5. Ley A, Jeffery DP, McLaren S, Siegfried N. *Psychosocial treatment programmes for people with both severe mental illness and substance misuse* (Cochrane Review). In: The Cochrane Library, Issue 2, 2003. Oxford: Update Software.
6. Johnson S. Dual diagnosis of severe mental illness and substance misuse: a case for specialist services? *British Journal of Psychiatry* 1997; 171: 205-8.
7. Kleber HD. Treatment of drug dependence: what works. *International Review of Psychiatry* 1989; 1: 81-100.
8. Crits-Christoph P, Siqueland L. Psychosocial treatment for drug abuse. *Archives of General Psychiatry* 1996; 53: 749-56.
9. American Psychiatric Association (1987), Diagnostic and statistical manual of mental disorders. III-R, edition, American Psychiatric Press, Washington DC, 1999.
10. Gerstein DR. *Outcome research: Drug Abuse.* In: Galanter M, Kleber HD, eds. Textbook of Substance Abuse Treatment. Washington DC: American Psychiatric Press, 2e ed: 135-47.
11. American Psychiatric Association Practice guideline for the treatment of patients with substance use disorders: alcohol, cocaine, opioids, in *American Journal of Psychiatry* 1995; 152 (suppl 11): 1-59.

Achevé d'imprimer par Corlet, Imprimeur, S.A.
14110 Condé-sur-Noireau
N° d'Imprimeur : 74012 - Dépôt légal : novembre 2003

Imprimé en France